MY BODY'S SUPERPOWER

MY BODY'S SUPERPOWER

THE GIRLS' GUIDE TO GROWING UP HEALTHY DURING PUBERTY

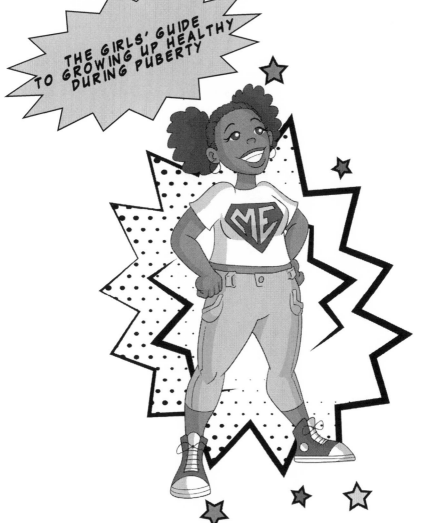

MARYANN JACOBSEN

ISBN 978-0-9995645-3-0

Library of Congress Control Number 2019937609

Cover Illustration by Hannah Patrico
Cover design and interior illustrations by Jeanine Henning, JH Illustrations
Book design by Maureen Cutajar, www.gopublished.com
Editing by Arnetta Jackson

First printing

Published by Jacobsen Publishing

MaryannJacobsen.com

JACOBSEN PUBLISHING

CONTENTS

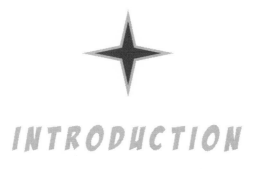

INTRODUCTION

FROM SECRET POWERS TO SUPERPOWERS

IMAGINE IF SUPERHEROES LIKE SUPERGIRL OR WONDER WOMAN never discovered their powers. Think how different the world would be. All those people wouldn't be saved and the bad guys would have won. And the superheroes themselves would be unhappy, feeling like something was missing in their lives.

Although superheroes aren't real, their stories tell an important truth you are about to discover. As you go through puberty and your body changes, you gain many superpowers. But unlike superheroes, your body's amazing abilities are less noticeable and often stay secret.

That's how it was for me growing up. I had no idea of my body's superpowers. It wasn't until I graduated high school that I became aware of a couple of them. But it took many years to discover–and use–them all. Too long, I say. But that's why I've written this book. I want things to be different for you, and every girl out there.

CHANGE IS COMING

I am a registered dietitian, mom, and author. I've written several books for parents about raising healthy children, but I decided it was now time to write for younger generations. That's because as you approach and get into double digits (10 and beyond!), you need to learn how to take care of your body. This stage of development is considered *early adolescence* and it signals a great amount of change coming.

> *Adolescence is the time period between puberty and adulthood. Early adolescence (10-14) is important for learning about your body because this is when the changes of puberty start. Figure things out now, and it will help you not just for the rest of adolescence, but for the rest of your life!*

You may be thinking, "I already know about healthy choices." But just knowing what to do does not make a person healthy. It's better to get to know your amazing body because it holds all the answers. That's why this book focuses on three steps to using and enjoying all of your body's superpowers. Let's take a look.

STEP #1: SUPER KNOWLEDGE

The first step is learning about all the changes going on inside you. Without this information, you may assume that something is wrong or even be scared. But I promise you, there is a reason for each and every change you experience. Without this knowledge your powers stay hidden and you are unable to fully use them. That's why I call it Super Knowledge—it gives your mind all the information it needs to open up to your Superpowers.

There are other books that talk about menstruating, hygiene, and how sex organs like your breasts change. This is not that kind of book. The purpose of this book is to help you understand your changing body so you can learn to take care of it. Only then can you master its superpowers and use them for a force for good in your life.

STEP #2: BODY TALK

After learning what's going on inside your body, you'll discover how your body talks to you. Learning its language is key to mastering each and every superpower. Whether it's your Appetite Signals, Internal Compass, or Super Functioning, listening closely is key. Unfortunately, many girls don't know how to listen to their body, so they miss these signals. But not anymore!

Like any first-rate superhero, you'll want to stick with the superpowers you have. I mean The Flash would probably love to fly like Supergirl, but that's not *his* superpower. He could work day and night trying to fly and make no progress—and end up feeling awful about himself. He'd be better off mastering his own superpowers—like moving at lightning speed!

One example of this is when puberty starts. You don't have the power to change that because it's mostly determined by your *genes*. You can work to speed up or slow down puberty but all it will do is frustrate you. By sticking to your superpower of X-ray Vision (being able to clearly see why things are the way they are), you will be happier and healthier.

STEP #3: TIME TRAVEL

If you are like most young people, you think about how you feel *right now*. And that can tempt you to go against your superpowers. This is where your power of Time Travel comes in. When making a decision, imagine yourself in the future and how you will feel then as a result of your decision. This can even be a few days ahead. So if you have homework over the weekend, imagine how you'll feel Sunday night if you decide to wait to do it then, rather than doing it now. It won't feel so hot then to have to skip family game night.

When you learn about and master your superpowers, your future self—which eventually catches up with you—is always better off. But it's not always easy to see that right now. Like any skill, mastering Time Travel takes time and practice.

Together, Super Knowledge, Body Talk, and Time Travel help you make Super Decisions. Check in with these three and you'll easily master your body's superpowers. This book will show you how!

THE SUPERPOWER FORMULA

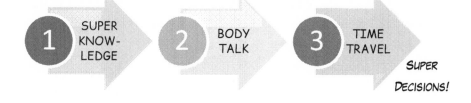

THE THREE TYPES OF SUPERPOWERS

This first part of the book focuses on your body's *physical powers*: how your body changes during puberty and what you can give it so it thrives. The second part focuses on your *emotional powers*, those sticky feelings, friendships, and how you feel about the type of person you are becoming. Last is your *outside powers* and how to use them with the pressures of both the virtual and real worlds.

You will be introduced to a total of nine of your body's superpowers which deliver super health, allowing you to live an amazing and full life. I call this My Body's Superpower because together these superpowers make up a miraculous force of health and happiness. Leave one out, and your body's superpower isn't as strong.

> PHYSICAL POWERS
> + EMOTIONAL POWERS
> + OUTSIDE POWERS
> = MY BODY'S SUPERPOWER

Each chapter ends with Super Decisions, stories that show how girls use their newfound knowledge, body communication, and Time Travel in different situations. Some of these are true stories but most of them are fictional examples. If you want to practice on your own, there's a journal that goes along with this book (or you can just use any journal to write in). And remember, mistakes are how you learn. All superheroes make mistakes and learn from them!

Oh, and one more thing. Almost every time you see a word italicized, it means it's included in the glossary at the back of the book with its meaning. You've got a lot of learning to do!

START DISCOVERING YOUR BODY'S SUPERPOWERS

Consider reading this book along with a trusted adult like your mom, aunt, grandmother, or family friend. Ask them how they felt during puberty, share your own worries, and you'll both learn a lot from each other. After all, every woman you know has gone through puberty and has wisdom to share. But if you don't feel comfortable doing this, that's okay too.

I hope you are ready to learn just how amazing your body is. Let's get started with the timing and physical changes that occur during puberty.

Consider yourself a Superhero in training!

PART 1

PHYSICAL POWERS

"YOU ARE STRONGER THAN YOU BELIEVE. YOU HAVE GREATER POWERS THAN YOU KNOW."
-ANTIOPE TO DIANA, *WONDER WOMAN* MOVIE

CHAPTER 1

X-RAY VISION

X-RAY VISION ALLOWS SUPERHEROES TO SEE WHAT OTHERS CAN'T see. Well, humans have X-ray Vision too. This is gaining knowledge about how your body is changing. Once you learn what you need to learn, you can see things much more clearly.

SUPER KNOWLEDGE: PUBERTY TIMING

So first things first. You need to understand the course of puberty and the growth that will happen. The more you understand, the better you can see!

THE START OF PUBERTY

When you were a baby you grew fast. This super speed growth slows down after age two and becomes more stable until you reach puberty. *Puberty* is the period of time the body gradually transforms from that of a child to an adult. Now, your body is going to be growing almost as fast as when you were a baby. But this growth spurt is two times longer. It's called the *adolescent growth spurt*.

You do not have control over when you start puberty—nobody does. This timing mostly has to do with your *genes,* which were transferred to you from your biological parents. Genes determine traits like hair color, height, eye color, and when you start puberty.

Puberty starts when a small but important part of the brain, the *hypothalamus,* provides a signal that it's time for the body to release hormones. *Hormones* are substances in your bloodstream that instruct other cells in your body to take action. In girls, the main hormone is called *estrogen* and in boys it's *testosterone.* For example, estrogen tells the female body to develop breasts and get ready for *menstruation* (also called a period).

Girls typically enter puberty around 10-11 and boys, 11-12. But there is a wide range for what is considered normal— anywhere between 8 and 14. Everyone is different. While one girl starts puberty at 9, another girl the same age may not start for another two years!

SUPER ADVICE

I felt like the last girl on earth to start puberty. Now I know that some girls feel like the first girl on earth, and some think it will never happen, or will never stop. But everyone who reaches adulthood goes through puberty. When a person will start puberty is determined the moment the sperm and ovum meet. All this to say, it will start when it's supposed to start, and will end when it's supposed to end. There is no right or wrong timeline.

—Marnie Goldenberg, Sex Education Specialist

How Puberty Progresses: (Years 1 & 2 after First Signs)

For girls, the first sign of puberty is breast development. This may start with some tenderness and the development of breast buds (raised bumps). Following breasts buds is the growth of *pubic hair*. That is the hair just above your vagina. It can occur during breast budding or a few weeks or even months later.

The first year or two following the first signs of puberty–breast buds and pubic hair–you can expect your breasts to become more full and your pubic hair to get darker and more coarse. You will also notice that you have some *vaginal discharge*–from white and cream-like to watery and clear–which is normal and shows up on your underwear.

In addition to pubic hair, hair on your legs and underarms will grow. You will also notice you sweat more, especially during physical activity or in the heat, and you might need more frequent showers and deodorant.

About one year after the first signs you will enter what is called your *peak growth period*. This is the time you grow fastest.

How Tall Will I Be?

Many girls want to know how tall they will be. Most likely your height will be similar to your parents because of that whole gene thing. While there is no way to know for sure, try this formula for fun. Add up your mother's and father's height in inches. Girls subtract 5 inches and boys add 5 inches and then divide by two. So to do it for a girl whose mom is 5'4" (64 inches) and dad is 6'1" (73 inches), that adds up to 137 inches and subtract 5 to equal 132. If you divide 132 by 2 you get 66 inches (5'6").

YOUR PERIOD (ABOUT 1-3 YEARS AFTER FIRST SIGNS)

Most girls will get their first period about two years after the first signs of puberty, but some may get it early (after 1 year) or late (year 4). The average age for starting menstruation is 12-13, but there is a wide range—anywhere from age 10 to 17.

Most girls stop growing around age 14-16, about two years after their periods start. This makes the total time of puberty around four years, sometimes shorter, sometimes longer. Other parts of your body will continue to grow, including your brain and bones. Table 1.1 summarizes the 5 stages of puberty.

TABLE 1.1: THE 5 STAGES OF PUBERTY

STAGE 1 PRE-ADOLESCENT	RIGHT BEFORE PUBERTY, NO SIGNS YET
STAGE 2	MY FIRST SIGNS ARE BREAST BUDDING AND PUBIC HAIR
STAGE 3	MY GROWTH IS AT FULL BLAST! BREASTS BECOME FULLER, PUBIC HAIR MORE COARSE, AND HAIR GROWS UNDER ARMS AND ON LEGS
STAGE 4	MY PERIOD STARTS. THIS IS ABOUT 2-2.5 YEARS AFTER FIRST SIGNS. GROWTH SLOWS DOWN
STAGE 5	MY BREASTS REACH ADULT SIZE. GROWTH STOPS AROUND 14-16 (ABOUT 4 YEARS AFTER FIRST SIGNS)

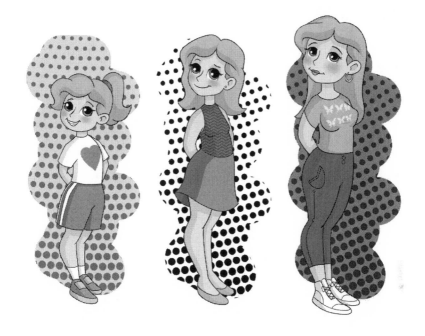

Body Talk: Weight Gain

Knowing what to expect during puberty helps sharpen your X-ray Vision abilities. Now it's time to decode the messages your body sends and respond to them. It's Body Talk time!

Fast Growth in Action

The first message your body sends to you is in the form of weight gain. Remember, this is faster than it was for as many years as you can remember (you probably don't remember growing fast as a baby, but I bet your parents do!). When you start gaining weight, do not fear; it goes along with puberty.

Table 1.2 shows you how much faster your growth is during puberty. You gain 2-4 times as much weight and your height rate can double. That is super growth!

TABLE 1.2: FROM STABLE TO SUPER GROWTH

	STABLE GROWTH PRESCHOOL TO SCHOOL AGE (AVERAGE)	SUPER GROWTH DURING PUBERTY (RANGES)
HEIGHT	2-2.5 INCHES/YEAR	2.4-4 INCHES/YEAR
WEIGHT	5 POUNDS/YEAR	12-23 POUNDS/YEAR

AN IMPORTANT PART OF WEIGHT GAIN: BODY FAT

Here's a secret: you need a certain amount of body fat to get your period, which is part of the weight you gain during puberty. Many girls tend to "fill out" before they grow up, initially gaining a layer of fat which may give them a rounded belly. In time, this fat around the middle is redistributed to the breasts, thighs, and hips to give you some curves.

Different than boys, girls' peak growth in both height and weight (around age 12) happens at different times, which can make it feel "out of proportion" until growth is complete. It's very important for you and your parents to understand what is happening so nobody panics or makes an issue of these changes in body shape.

SUPER TIP!

Fat is not a bad word! While you may hear people say "fat" as a negative way of describing bodies, your Super X-ray Vision sees something different. Fat is actually a healthy part of every body, especially in girls during puberty. Without it we wouldn't get to the next stage in life, or even be born. Isn't it amazing what the body can do? Thank you, fat!

A WORD ABOUT BOYS

During puberty boys' body changes are different than yours. For example, boys gain more muscle than fat. But their peak growth period (around 14) occurs later in puberty than girls and they keep growing until about age 18-19. By the late teens, boys have about half the body fat girls have and are typically taller.

Table 1.3 summarizes the key differences between boys and girls during puberty. Some boys may not noticeably grow until late in high school, which can make them feel self-conscious.

TABLE 1.3: THE DIFFERENCE BETWEEN BOYS & GIRLS

GIRLS	BOYS
START PUBERTY AROUND 10-11	START PUBERTY AROUND 11-12
PEAK GROWTH OCCURS EARLY IN PUBERTY	PEAK GROWTH OCCURS LATER IN PUBERTY
PUBERTY LASTS ON AVERAGE ABOUT 4 YEARS	PUBERTY LASTS ON AVERAGE ABOUT 6 YEARS
GIRLS GAIN FAT AND MUSCLE DURING PUBERTY	BOYS GAIN MORE MUSCLE THAN FAT DURING PUBERTY

YOUR BONES, MUSCLES, AND BLOOD GROW TOO

Did you know that bone is a living tissue that grows and expands throughout your childhood? Your bones grow relatively slow until the super growth phase of puberty. The peak in bone growth occurs around 12.5 years for girls and 14 years for boys. Ninety-five percent of your adult bone mass is reached about four years after this peak.

Your body doesn't really send you messages unless something goes wrong. When your bones are growing they first grow wider followed by deposits of calcium to make them more solid and strong. This temporary gap before the achievement of *peak bone mass* puts you at higher risk for fractures than adults.

During puberty your muscles increase both in size and fiber thickness, boosting your ability to get physically stronger. With changes in your muscle, body fat, and bones, you also have more blood circulating around your body. Growing tissues during puberty need more oxygen and nutrients which are delivered in the blood.

SUPER TIP!

Your X-ray Vision shows you how important your bones are, so take care of them. About half of boys and a third of girls will sustain a fracture by the time they turn 18.

ACCEPTANCE AND ADVANTAGE

Your X-ray Vision helps you see that the growth and weight gain you experience during puberty is normal and is to be expected. How do you talk back when your body is talking to you? This is where the two A's can help.

Acceptance is choosing not to fight something, like bodily changes during puberty. It's okay to have mixed feelings about them, but spending time trying to change it isn't the best use of time.

The other A is Advantage, using where you are to your advantage in some way. For instance, early puberty means muscles grow sooner and perhaps give you an advantage in sports. And late puberty means you don't have to worry about your periods for a while. You may not be able to change when puberty starts, but you can always find something positive about it. Time Travel helps too.

TIME TRAVEL

Looking into your future can help in many ways. First, eventually the out-of-proportion growth you are experiencing will end as you move farther along through puberty. And wherever you are on your puberty journey won't matter so much, as girls (and eventually boys) will catch up in high school. Ask the adult women in your life when they went through puberty and you will hear a variety of stories. But all went through it at different times and now don't think much about it.

SUPER DECISIONS: YOUR X-RAY VISION IN ACTION

Let's put everything you learned together: Your Super Knowledge about puberty timing, your superpower Body Talk (which includes weight gain), and your Time Travel skills.

WHEN PUBERTY IS EARLY

Emily started puberty early and felt self conscious of her growing body. She was the only one she knew who got her period in the 5th grade. One time her maxi pad fell out of her backpack and her teacher asked the whole class whose it was. "I was quite embarrassed, so I didn't speak up," she said. "I was surprised she expected someone to step forward. It was hard to be the first one to go through all of these changes, and this didn't help."

Going through puberty early can be challenging for girls. If you fall into this category, remember that girls get it early based on genes so it's no one's fault. Also, some Time Travel to the future shows you that everyone else will catch up to you by middle school or high school at the latest. This "only me" phase won't last forever.

Last, girls who start puberty younger gain certain superpowers earlier such as developing muscle and strength, which helps with sports. Instead of fighting these changes, it makes sense to accept them and take advantage of your timing.

WHEN PUBERTY IS LATE

Amy had the opposite problem from Emily, meaning she was late to start puberty. Most of the girls in her 7th grade class had started developing; and strangers thought she was still in elementary school.

Amy mastered her X-ray Vision by learning about puberty timing and talking to her mom, who also went through puberty late. Time Travel to the future reminded her that by high school she'd catch up; and in the meantime, she didn't have to worry about her periods. Because her superpowers couldn't change when puberty came, she focused on the joys of being a child while she could. Sure enough, by summer she got her first signs of puberty and got her period by the end of her first year of high school.

FROM X-RAY VISION TO APPETITE SIGNALS

X-ray Vision is learning about the changes going on in your body and accepting and using them to your advantage. It's one of the most important superpowers you have.

Now it's time to add another powerful one: Appetite Signals. With all this growth, you will get hungrier than usual. It's the perfect time to master this amazing superpower.

CHAPTER 2

APPETITE SIGNALS

APPETITE IS YOUR BASIC DESIRE TO EAT TO SATISFY YOUR BODY'S hunger signals. During puberty these signals can be especially loud. Learn to use them now, and it will make getting the right amount of food for you "easy peasy."

SUPER KNOWLEDGE: THE GROWTH APPETITE CONNECTION

The first task is teaching you how appetite is related to growth, which includes body shape and size. And of course, genes matter too.

THE FOUR APPETITE SIGNALS

During puberty your appetite is high because it needs more food for your super growth. The first body signal is *hunger*. Your brain releases the hormone *ghrelin* to signal it's time to eat. Your stomach makes rumbling noises. When the body has had enough food, the brain releases another hormone called *leptin*. This tells your stomach to send *fullness* signals. Appetite signal number two is *fullness*, when your stomach extends and feels full of food.

Two other less-talked about signals are *satisfaction* and *craving*. Satisfaction is how much you enjoy a meal and craving is when you desire to eat a certain type of food. All of these Appetite Signals influence each other. For example, if you're not enjoying a meal, you may not eat until fullness. Or if you have a craving, once you get to eat the desired food, you might eat past fullness.

It's important to listen to all these signals because they are your body's way of telling you how much food you need to grow up healthy. Everyone has a different appetite and that's okay. Some people need more food than others. And everyone enjoys and craves different foods. Most girls going through puberty get hungrier, and that's totally normal and to be expected. Table 2.1 summarizes the four Appetite Signals.

TABLE 2.1: APPETITE SIGNALS

APPETITE SIGNAL	WHAT IT FEELS LIKE	WHY IT'S IMPORTANT
HUNGER	MY STOMACH RUMBLES AND FEELS EMPTY	YOUR BODY'S WAY OF TELLING YOU IT NEEDS FOOD
FULLNESS	MY STOMACH FEELS FULL OF FOOD	YOUR BODY'S WAY OF TELLING YOU IT'S HAD ENOUGH
SATISFACTION	I'M REALLY ENJOYING THIS MEAL/FOOD; I'M DONE AND DON'T WANT MORE	ENJOYMENT ENSURES THAT YOU EAT ENOUGH
CRAVING	I WANT ONE TYPE OF FOOD REALLY BAD	YOUR BODY'S TELLING YOU SOMETHING; IF THE FEELING IS SUPPRESSED, CRAVINGS MAY INCREASE

GROWTH, SHAPE, AND SIZE

Although Appetite Signals impact growth, so do your genes. Your body has a *genetic blueprint* handed down from your parents. This is the general frame and shape it will be after you are done growing. Bodies come in a variety of sizes and shapes.

Ten-year-old Suzi has parents that are short and thin, so it's no surprise that Suzy will become an adult who also has a small frame. Eleven-year-old Sherry has an athletic build—muscular with broad shoulders—as does many of her family members. Bodies come in many sizes, just like the picture shows.

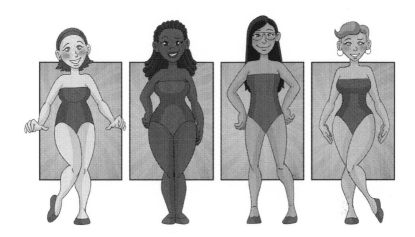

Let's consider body shape. When Suzi is done growing, she will have more of a rectangle shape, meaning her body will be more straight than curvy. Sherry, on the other hand, will have an apple shape which means her shoulders and chest are broader than her hips. Some teens and young adults have more of a pear shape which is when the hips are larger than the bust. Finally, there is an hourglass shape which is a narrow waist with hip and bust measurements more equal.

The figure below shows some examples; but no one fits each of these exactly. It just shows that shape and size varies from person to person.

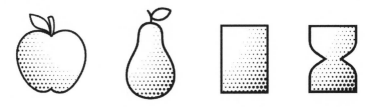

Choosing Superpowers That Work

It's normal not to love everything about your changing body. Maybe you're short and want to be tall or you have muscular arms and want them to look more delicate. Some people may stop listening to their Appetite Signals in order to change their body, which is referred to as *dieting*. It might be by eating less (not listening to hunger or reaching fullness), eating certain foods (forget satisfaction), or cutting items out (so long food cravings!).

But then your Appetite Signals get so loud they turn into alarms. So if you stop listening to hunger, one day your body can't take it anymore and the hunger alarm is so loud you eat until you get a bellyache. Or you cut out sugar and once you eat something sweet you feel like you can't stop. After all, you're fighting against your body's natural appetite and genes!

Changing your body is not a superpower you have; but honoring your body's Appetite Signals is. Plus, how do you think your body feels when you don't listen to it?

Some girls stop listening to their body's Appetite Signals because they are encouraged to. It could be a coach telling you to stop eating after dinner or a teacher saying sugar is bad. Always pause before taking advice and ask why they are offering it. Is it to get you stronger, fitter, or healthier? You can let them know you will take it under consideration, then talk to a parent or trusted adult. Just remember that ignoring your Appetite Signals almost never results in positive, long-term outcomes. Always work with your appetite instead of against it!

BODY TALK: CAN YOU HEAR THE SIGNAL?

Now that you've learned about your appetite signals, it's time to learn how to respond to the messages your body sends you about your appetite.

HOW TO RATE HUNGER AND FULLNESS

Your body sends you messages about how much food to eat. Hunger tells you how much to start with and fullness is your key to stopping. For example, before serving yourself food, consider where you are on a scale from 1-5 (1 being 'hangry,' and 5 past full). Is your hunger a 1, or 2? That can make the difference in how much food you take. Also, listen to the messages you get when you're eating. Stopping at 4 saves you from the uncomfortable feeling you get when eating past fullness. Table 2.2 summarizes hunger and fullness ratings.

TABLE 2.2: HUNGER AND FULLNESS RATINGS

1	**HANGRY!** BAD MOOD, TIRED, NAUSEATED, WANT TO EAT ANYTHING
2	**HUNGRY:** STOMACH GETTING EMPTY; FOOD SOUNDS GOOD
3	**HUNGER GONE:** EATEN ENOUGH, BUT NOT FULLY SATISFIED/FULL
4	**FULL:** SATISFIED AND COMFORTABLY FULL
5	**PAST FULL:** UNCOMFORTABLY FULL STOMACH; MAY START ACHING/FEEL EXTENDED

There are ways to help your hunger and fullness signals from getting too loud. First is planning regular meals and snacks so you don't go too long without eating. This keeps your hunger from dipping to a 1. Also, pay attention when you eat. If you do other things while eating, it's hard for this superpower to work. For example, you are so into your favorite TV show that you don't even remember eating all the popcorn.

Remember that mistakes are how you learn. Eleven-year-old Jane was so excited to have a root beer float that she drank it so quickly she almost threw up. She remembered that next time, and drank it slowly, listening to her body.

SUPER ADVICE

One thing I wish I had known during puberty was that of course I would be hungry after school, and having a snack was just fine (especially when I was minimizing lunches and playing

> *sports). Basically, knowing that being hungry was "okay" (and thus, eating was "okay") would have made getting the right amount of food easier because, I felt like I was "sneaking" food for snacks and I think that made me eat more than my body needed.*
>
> — *Jennifer Schmitt, mom of two girls*

SUPER FILLING FOODS

Some foods keep you full longer than others. Maybe you notice after having cereal in the morning you're hungry an hour later, but when you have an egg sandwich, you aren't hungry for about 3 hours. It's normal to be hungrier during puberty, but if you're hungry 24/7, it might be because of the type or combination of food you're choosing.

You can experiment with different foods to see what fills you up. Try adding foods with filling fiber like fruits, vegetables, beans, and whole grains. Protein foods like deli meat, eggs, cheese, beans, and tofu can also increase the filling factor. And adding a little satisfying fat to some foods makes a difference, such as sliced avocados to a sandwich, or nuts and seeds to cereal or yogurt. But everyone is different so just be aware of what foods and combination of foods provide lasting fullness for you. See Table 2.3 for some ideas on how to make snacks and meals more filling.

TABLE 2.3: MAKE IT MORE FILLING

BEFORE	AFTER
CRACKERS FOR SNACK	CRACKERS WITH SOME CHEESE AND AN APPLE

COLD CEREAL IN THE MORNING	CEREAL WITH NUTS AND DRIED FRUIT
TURKEY SANDWICH WITH MAYO	TURKEY SANDWICH WITH MAYO WITH LETTUCE AND TOMATO, AND WITH SOME BEAN SOUP OR GREEN SALAD

THE ENJOYMENT FACTOR

When meal satisfaction is high you enjoy what you are eating, and when you are done you aren't secretly longing to eat more. When meal satisfaction is low, you may never reach satisfied, even though you get full. To increase satisfaction, work with the main cook in the house. It's a great time for you to learn more about cooking and discover ways to make food tasty. By helping, you can influence the menu, learn new skills, and give the cook a break (all cooks need breaks!).

Cravings get a bad rap. It's important not to fight them; instead, be curious about them. For instance, if you start craving sweets all the time, it could be that you aren't getting enough sleep and activity. Or you may be stressed and looking for a distraction. Superpowers 4 and 5 can help with that. Most of the time, cravings are simply a desire to eat an enjoyable food. Talk to your parents about the foods you crave and make a plan for how to include them in a balanced way.

SUPER TIP!

Try different sauces, dips, and food combinations, and you might just find something you didn't like before is now one of your favorites.

TIME TRAVEL

Let's Time Travel to the future. If you stop listening to your Appetite Signals, they can turn into alarms that are hard to ignore. Sometimes your body grows faster or slower than it's meant to grow. This interferes with your life as you think about food all the time. In other words, you are taking over your body's job of deciding how much to eat when your body is better at it than you (or anybody else!). It's like the case of The Flash trying to fly like Supergirl, remember?

But let's say you stay the course and trust your body. Now and in the future, eating the amount your body needs is easy. You grow the way your body was meant to grow and you don't think about food all the time. Your Appetite Signals don't turn into annoying alarms and you feel good about your body. Plus, who knows how your unique body will help you in the future? Table 2.4 summarizes the benefits of trusting your body.

TABLE 2.4: TRUSTING YOUR BODY

NO TRUST; YOU WANT TO CHANGE	TRUST; YOU'RE GOOD!
MY BODY IS ALL WRONG AND I WILL TRY TO CHANGE IT BY IGNORING ITS SIGNALS OF HUNGER, FULLNESS, SATISFACTION, AND CRAVINGS (SKIPPING MEALS, EATING LESS, FOLLOWING A "DIET," CUTTING FOOD OUT).	I TRUST MY BODY AND RESPOND TO ITS APPETITE SIGNALS OF HUNGER, FULLNESS, SATISFACTION, AND CRAVINGS. THIS HELPS GIVE MY BODY WHAT IT NEEDS TO BE AT ITS BEST.

APPETITE SIGNALS TURN INTO ALARMS AND INTERFERE WITH LIFE. YOU SPEND TOO MUCH OF YOUR TIME THINKING ABOUT FOOD AND YOUR BODY. GROWTH MAY SPEED UP OR SLOW DOWN.

APPETITE SIGNALS DON'T TURN INTO ALARMS AND EATING IS ENJOYABLE AND EASY. THE BODY GROWS THE WAY IT'S SUPPOSED TO AND IT FEELS GOOD.

SUPER DECISIONS: APPETITE SIGNALS IN ACTION

Sometimes listening and honoring Appetite Signals gets tricky. Let's use a couple of examples to see how to use this superpower.

EMBRACING YOUR BODY BETTER IN THE LONG RUN

Maddy wanted to be more slender like the girls at her school. She would try to exercise, eat certain foods, and cut out sugar. "I try, and it always ends up not working," she said. "I wanted to be like everyone else, thin and fit, but it just never works!"

This is a case of trying to use a superpower you don't have. A sure sign this is happening is it's hard, takes a lot of energy, and it doesn't even work! Instead of trying to change your body, listen and trust its Appetite Signals. They make eating so easy! Use Time Travel to consider all the ways your body will be a force for good in the future. Olympic gold medalist Aly Raisman was made fun of for her muscular arms in middle school. But she trusted her body, which eventually became an asset. On her Instagram account she wrote:

Shoutout to all the boys from 5th-9th grade who made fun of me for being "too strong." Thanks for forcing me to learn to love myself and my body. My muscular arms that were considered weird and gross when I was younger have made me one of the best gymnasts on the planet. Don't ever let anyone tell you how you should or shouldn't look. There is no such thing as a perfect body type.

Not Satisfied

Since Julie can remember, people have been trying to get her to eat. Being thin with a small appetite worried those around her. As Julie hit puberty her hunger increased, but she didn't love all the meals her mom made. To get out of eating, she would say she was full but then later, when her parents weren't around, she'd head to the snack drawer.

Super Knowledge helped Julie understand that there was nothing wrong with her body and her Appetite Signals were important. Time Travel showed her that fibbing about being full would be too hard to keep up and would limit her relationship with her family. Rather than saying she was full to get out of meals, she worked with her mom to make meals more satisfying. They decided to take a cooking class together and it was so much fun! Soon, meals were more satisfying and she was branching out with food.

No matter what you do, enjoying your meals will help you get enough to eat and not worry about being hungry an hour after eating.

From Appetite Signals to Super Functioning

Appetite Signals are about trusting your body's signals for food and giving it what it needs to grow the way nature intended. That makes for a happy body!

Now let's move on to the types of food you consume by delving into superpower #3: Super Functioning.

CHAPTER 3

SUPER FUNCTIONING

EVERYONE LIKES TO EAT TASTY FOOD. BUT DID YOU KNOW FOOD'S job has just begun after you eat it? That's because your body needs food to function. And during puberty when growth is high, nutrition needs are high too. Super Functioning helps your body run in tip-top shape during puberty and beyond!

SUPER KNOWLEDGE: HOW YOUR BODY USES FOOD

Let's get into the nitty-gritty about how your body uses food to do its various jobs.

FROM FOOD TO NUTRIENTS

When you travel somewhere there is a process. You pack clothes, get in a car or on a plane, and finally make it to your destination. When you eat food there's a traveling process too. After it's chewed and swallowed, food travels down your esophagus to your stomach and is released to your small and large intestines. And guess where the final destination is? The toilet! That's when you poop it out!

Your *digestive system* breaks food down into nutrients so your body can use it. There are big nutrients, called *macronutrients* and small nutrients called *micronutrients*. Macronutrients provide *energy*, often called *calories*, and include *carbohydrates, protein*, and *fat*. Micronutrients don't provide energy but they do important work inside your body. They are called *vitamins* and *minerals*.

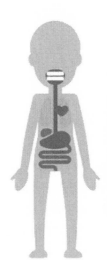

Digestive System
The first stop for your food is your digestive system, which breaks food down. When food is digested, fiber helps it move through faster. Probiotics, found in fermented foods like yogurt, provide good bacteria, and water helps keep your gastrointestinal tract healthy.

NUTRIENTS GO TO WORK IN THE BODY

The body has many nutrient "worker bees." After food is broken down from the digestive system, nutrients are *absorbed* into the blood and travel to different parts of your body. Your *circulatory system* makes this possible. Basically, your heart pumps nutrient- and oxygen-rich blood through arteries and veins. With rapid growth during puberty, your blood volume increases to meet these demands.

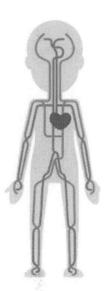

Circulatory System

The mineral iron ensures all the cells in your body get enough oxygen from the air you breathe. The minerals magnesium and potassium work with blood vessels and the heart to pump blood throughout the body.

One of the first places nutrients go is to your *nervous system* which consists of the brain, spinal cord, and nerves. The circulatory system knows the brain is a priority and rushes nutrients to it. It's the big boss of the nervous system, sending it messages about what to do. These messages travel from the brain to the spinal cord, which contain small, delicate nerves (like a thread) that can reach every part of the body.

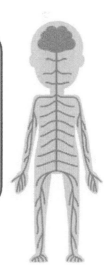

Nervous System

Your brain requires constant energy from carbohydrates. DHA, a fat found primarily in fish, is stored in the brain. Having enough of this type of fat stored helps as the structure of your brain changes during puberty, allowing for better thinking, learning, and creativity.

Your *skeletal system* is like the foundation used to make a house—it supports your body's structure. The *exoskeleton* is the outer shell and the *endoskeleton* supports the body internally. Both types are comprised of bones that are growing, expanding, and becoming more dense during puberty. How strong your bones grow now affects how strong they will be when you get older (that's some major Time Travel, but you can do it!).

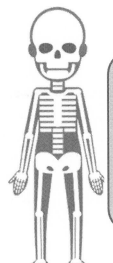

Skeletal System
The mineral Calcium is deposited into your bones to make them strong. Vitamin D has many jobs in your body, but it's best known for ensuring calcium gets into your bones. Physical activity also helps your bones grow strong.

Your *muscular system* allows your body to move. Skeletal muscles are attached to your bones and involve voluntary movement like walking and throwing a ball. During puberty, these muscles grow both in size and fiber strength. Together with the skeletal system, these muscles form another system called the *musculoskeletal system*.

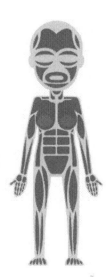

Muscular System

To grow strong muscles during puberty your body needs enough energy from carbohydrates, protein, and fat. Protein is especially important and so is the mineral zinc. And of course, physical activity helps your muscles grow and develop.

The *integumentary system* includes your skin, hair, nails, and sweat. Skin protects your body by keeping harmful substances from entering. Hair and skin are modified versions of skin, but once they grow they are no longer living tissue. Hair covers and protects most of the body. Nails grow and protect fingers and toes. Sweat, on the other hand, helps the body regulate temperature by cooling it off when it gets too hot.

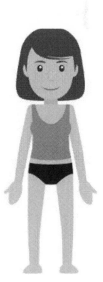

Integumentary System

Vitamin C is a key worker for your skin. It helps make collagen, a component of skin. That being said, the skin has a whole team of workers as it's your body's protective layer preventing harmful substances from entering.

While I highlighted specific nutrients, many different nutrients from food work to keep your body strong and healthy. Let's see which foods they are hiding in!

FROM NUTRIENTS TO FOOD

We don't eat nutrients, we eat food (which contains the nutrients). To make nutritious eating easier, experts categorize food together into food groups based on similar nutrition. For example, many fruits contain carbohydrates, fiber, and vitamin C, while vegetables tend to have fiber and vitamin A. Dairy foods and nondairy alternatives like soy and almond milk, tend to be good sources of calcium and vitamin D. Meat, beans, fish, and nuts have protein and iron, and grains have carbohydrates, fiber (whole grains), and B vitamins.

The first step is familiarizing yourself with food groups, as seen in Table 3.1. Do you eat from all the food groups, or is there some you skimp on?

TABLE 3.1: FOOD GROUPS

FOOD GROUP	FOOD TYPE
FRUITS	APPLES, PEARS, BANANAS, BLUEBERRIES, RASPBERRIES, HONEYDEW, WATERMELON, GRAPEFRUIT, GRAPES, PRUNES, PLUMS, DRIED FRUIT
VEGETABLES	CARROTS, CAULIFLOWER, BRUSSELS SPROUTS, SWEET POTATO, CUCUMBER, ZUCCHINI, SQUASH, MUSHROOMS, TOMATOES, GREEN BEANS, SUGAR SNAP PEAS, CELERY

GRAINS	WHITE: WHITE BREAD, WHITE RICE, BAGELS, CRACKERS, PRETZELS, AND PASTA WHOLE GRAINS: OATS SUCH AS OATMEAL, POPCORN, CRACKERS, WHOLE CORN, WHOLE GRAIN PRETZELS, PASTA AND BREAD, BROWN RICE, QUINOA
DAIRY AND NONDAIRY SOURCES OF CALCIUM	MILK, CHEESE, YOGURT, COTTAGE CHEESE, NON-DAIRY ALTERNATIVES SUCH AS SOY, ALMOND, AND RICE MILK
PROTEIN FOODS	ANIMAL SOURCES: MEAT (BEEF, PORK, CHICKEN, ETC.), FISH, AND SHELLFISH PLANT SOURCES: BEANS, SOY, NUTS, AND SEEDS
FAT SOURCES	OILS, BUTTER, AVOCADO, NUTS, SEEDS, AND NUT BUTTERS

BODY TALK: WHAT SUPER FUNCTIONING FEELS LIKE

Your body talks to you about how it is running. Let's find out what it says and how to give your body what it needs to maximize Super Functioning!

BODY SYSTEM TALK (AND WHEN YOU GET THE SILENT TREATMENT)

One of the loudest messages your body sends comes straight from your digestive system. If your poops are hard or infrequent, and if you have recurrent stomachaches or diarrhea, you may not be getting enough fiber or water to move things along. On the other hand, when your poop is regular, soft, and formed, this is a Super Functioning sign!

If your blood becomes low in iron, your body may start to feel tired. If it gets worse, you will get even more tired, pale, and may experience headaches. These are symptoms of iron deficiency anemia, the most common anemia. When you have enough iron in your blood, you won't feel tired (unless you don't get enough sleep) and you can concentrate better.

When the brain lacks a steady source of carbohydrates (in the form of broken down glucose), it has trouble paying attention, learning, and may feel low on energy. If your skin, hair, and nails don't look healthy, you may be lacking nutrients. A nutritious, colorful diet with enough energy helps your skin look rosy and your hair and nails grow strong. See table 3.2 for some examples of super versus reduced functioning.

TABLE 3.2: FUNCTIONING DIFFERENCES

SUPER FUNCTIONING	REDUCED FUNCTIONING
YOU FEEL ENERGIZED AND READY FOR ANYTHING. YOU CAN PAY ATTENTION AND AREN'T DISTRACTED.	YOU FEEL LOW ON ENERGY AND HAVE TROUBLE PAYING ATTENTION. YOU FEEL DISTRACTED.
YOU HAVE SOFT POOPS, IT'S EASY TO GO, AND YOU GO DAILY OR EVERY OTHER DAY.	YOU HAVE INFREQUENT POOPS THAT MAY BE HARD TO PASS. YOU MAY HAVE STOMACHACHES, GAS, AND OCCASIONAL DIARRHEA.

| YOUR SKIN IS GLOWING, YOUR HAIR IS SHINY, YOUR NAILS ARE STRONG AND GROW EASILY. | YOUR SKIN DOESN'T HAVE THAT GLOW, YOUR HAIR IS NOT SHINY, AND NAILS MAY NOT GROW AS WELL OR THEY BREAK OFF EASILY. |

DON'T FORGET WATER!

Your body is 50-60% water! Water regulates body temperature, flushes waste, acts as a shock absorber for the brain and spinal cord, helps convert food into energy, and is a major component of blood, muscle, brain, and even bones. You may find you are more thirsty during puberty as you grow faster. Try to always have water on hand to answer the call of your body!

SUPER FOOD

Before we go into eating advice, you need to know these are *guidelines*, not rules. Eating patterns—how you eat over time—matters more than any single food. If you don't like fruit, for example, don't beat yourself up. If your family has a limited budget and you can only follow these guidelines a couple of times a week, that's to be celebrated. It's the long game that matters.

So when someone says eating something is "good" or "bad" for you, that's not what we are aiming for. It's the pattern of eating you want for more energy and a healthy body. Removing good, bad, healthy, and unhealthy from your food vocabulary is empowering. The SUPER acronym can help you work on your pattern of eating so you get the nutrition you need.

Stick with fruits and vegetables at most meals and snacks. They contain fiber, vitamins C and A (and others), and potassium. They are crunchy and make a great addition to any meal or snack.

Up the amount of calcium-rich foods where you can. This includes dairy and nondairy alternatives. (See back of the book for a full list of calcium foods.) Eat three or four times daily to help build strong, growing bones. Also look for vitamin D, which are in many of these foods.

Pick whole grains half the time. These are unrefined grains such as oats, whole wheat bread, brown rice, and quinoa. They contain fiber, iron, and magnesium.

Eat fats too. Especially plant fat sources such as nuts and seeds, nut butters, avocado, and olive oil as they contain magnesium, vitamin E, and other minerals your body needs.

Realize the power of protein. Round out meals with a protein source. Aim to include fish and beans a couple of times a week. Fatty fish like salmon and tuna contain DHA and vitamin D; and beans are rich in fiber, potassium, iron, and many other nutrients.

When you fall short on certain food groups due a food allergy/intolerance, dislikes, or choosing to be *vegetarian,* talk to a trusted adult about taking dietary supplements or buying fortified foods. *Dietary supplements* are pills (can be chewable) that add nutrients you can't get in your diet. Some foods already have extra nutrients built in to help you get more through the foods you eat.

HELLO TASTE, MEET NUTRITION

Do you remember the importance of satisfaction and food cravings when using your Appetite Signals? Well, they matter for Super Functioning too. When you enjoy a meal, your digestive system works better, meaning more nutrients get into your blood. So you need to find a way to combine enjoyment with nutrition. But this is a skill that takes time to master.

For example, instead of eating tortilla chips alone, you make them into nachos by adding melted cheese and beans (or any other protein source). If you are ordering out and are getting something deep fried like chicken fingers, you opt for the seasonal fresh fruit as a side, instead of fries (which are also deep fried). The bonus is you get tasty and nutritious fruit minus the stomachache you might get from too much fat at a meal. Fried foods are rich in fat and low in fiber, so they can just sit in your stomach, instead of passing through your digestive system right away. You can save the fries for the next time you order a main meal that isn't fried.

Your amazing body can help you learn how all your favorite foods fit in. If you eat a bunch of cookies and nothing else, you may feel a bit sick. If you eat cookies as part of a meal, they may be the perfect finish. Considering nutrition and taste in addition to Super Functioning is the winning combination! I call this balance.

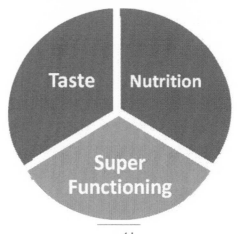

Time Travel

Time Travel is important for Super Functioning because what you do today can affect your body later. For example, you won't feel a difference right now from not getting enough calcium, but in your future, your bones may not be as strong. Also, finding tasty ways to include a variety of nutritious foods now will make it easier when you are an adult. Learning to like a variety of food takes time, many tastes, and experimentation. Like anything, it's easier to learn during childhood than as an adult. See the back of the book for some recipe and food ideas.

Super Decisions: Super Functioning in Action

Let's see how to use the Super Functioning superpower with all the challenges tweens and teens like you face.

Not Considering Nutrition

Twelve-year-old Emma knew about nutrition but didn't care much about it. When she sat down to eat, she wanted to enjoy her food. This caused friction because her mom cared a lot about nutrition. It seemed everything Emma liked wasn't considered "healthy enough" by her mom. When she was at her friend's house she ate as much candy as she could. She often felt constipated and sluggish.

Emma gained Super Knowledge about what her body needed to run efficiently. Time Travel told her that she'd want to stay healthy, especially in college where she planned to play soccer. She also noticed how her energy was often low, affecting her performance. She made the decision to be more open to eating nutritious foods by finding new ways to make them taste delicious.

She was able to add more fruits to her meals and discovered how great roasted vegetables taste, which helped her digestive system. She even created her very own pre-exercise trail mix which had cereal, nuts, dried fruit, and chocolate chips. And she didn't have to give up her favorite candy; but now she didn't want to eat it all the time, like before.

CALCIUM WOES

Jenna didn't like milk or cheese, and only took a bite or two of yogurt. Now that she was going through puberty her calcium needs went up and she understood how important it was for her growing bones. She used Time Travel to look into her future and definitely wanted strong bones later in life!

Jenna discovered all the different sources of calcium. She found ways to eat some dairy in homemade hot chocolate and smoothies. She tried a bunch of different yogurts to find one she really liked and added granola and chocolate chips to it. She started to include calcium-fortified cereals and orange juice, hard cheeses like parmesan, green leafy vegetables, and almonds. Not only was she able to get more calcium, she also added more enjoyment and variety to her diet.

FROM SUPER FUNCTIONING TO SUPER FOCUS

Super Functioning is learning what your body needs during the adolescent growth spurt and applying nutrition into your eating so it's enjoyable and you feel great. It helps you do everything better!

Now, let's discover the power that moving and resting your body has on how you feel, learn, and remember every single day! It's your Super Focus!

CHAPTER 4

SUPER FOCUS

ANOTHER VITAL PART OF YOUR PHYSICAL POWERS IS SUPER FOCUS. This means being able to concentrate and have a clear mind. And it boils down to two important behaviors: moving your body and resting it. This is often referred to as exercise and sleep (those aren't superpower words, but I'll use them for now).

SUPER KNOWLEDGE: YOUR MIND'S HELPERS

At a time when you really need it, you have two key helpers at your disposal. Exercise and sleep help your mind in amazing ways. Let's learn more.

HOW EXERCISE AND SLEEP HELP

Sleep and exercise help your entire body, not just your mind. For instance, exercise is crucial for your circulatory system because it makes your heart strong and healthy. It does wonders for your skeletal system because it helps build strong bones. It also benefits your muscular system by increasing muscle mass.

Exercise also helps you sleep better. And you need sleep! In fact, for puberty to go as planned, you need to be able to sleep deeply. This is when *luteinizing hormone* is released that sets all the changes into place. Also, hormones that help you grow are highest when you sleep. You need these hormones to get taller and change to your potential.

Super Tip!

Get your REM! An important type of sleep you need is called REM (rapid eye movement). This is a deeper type of sleep needed for growth and it is also when you dream. Some experts think that dreaming is your mind's way of reflecting and working out problems. Don't worry if you don't remember your dreams; many people don't.

Exercise and sleep also boost your mind and mood. Exercise increases blood flow to the brain and has been shown to help with mood, achievement, and stress level. And during sleep your brain moves what you learned that day to longer-term storage from a place called the *hippocampus* to the *cortex*.

When you wake up from a good night's sleep your mind is clear, and you're ready to learn even more the next day. So staying up late to study for that test—not such a great idea!

Sleep
- Clears the mind to optimize learning
- Helps mood
- Body feels energized

Activity
- Enhances learning and paying attention
- Improves mood
- Deeper sleep

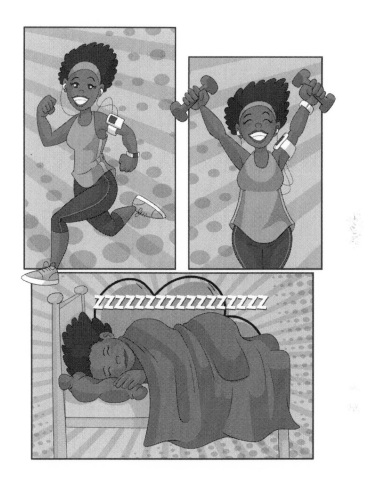

WHAT KEEPS THESE POWERS HIDDEN

Your sleep patterns change during puberty. Around the age 12 —
though the change is often gradual — your internal clock, called
circadian rhythm, shifts by a couple of hours. Your body delays the
release of the sleep hormone *melatonin.* Basically, you get tired
later and sleep in later than you used to.

Many tween and teen girls move their body less with all they have to do for school such as homework and projects. It's also a time some kids stop sports and get their first smart phone. What can make matters worse is nighttime device use, which delays the release of melatonin even more! There are also early school start times, after-school activities, and a growing list of to-dos.

These changes mean physical activity and sleep aren't maximized. No, they are hidden at a time girls need them most!

MANAGE SCREENS!

When screen time replaces sleep and physical activity, it becomes a problem. In fact, too much screen time depletes energy reserves, making exercise less likely. And staying up playing with devices means less sleep. Work with your parents on effective ways to structure screen time so it doesn't get in the way of your health and well being. For example, turn in your phone before going to bed.

JUST BECAUSE YOU CAN, DOESN'T MEAN YOU SHOULD

Bodies were designed to move and rest. For most of human history, walking was the main mode of transportation. Sleep wasn't a problem either because people went to bed when the sun went down and got up when the sun rose. There were no lights or devices to keep people up.

Just because we have the choice to stay up late and to not move much, doesn't mean we should make those choices. Knowing how much you need of these two helpers is the first step to uncovering their powers. Most tweens and teens need about an hour a day of exercise. It's totally okay to split this up and have days you get more and days you get less. You can also try to fit in a few days a week of activities that help build strong bones (jumping rope, etc.) and strengthen your muscles.

If you're between the ages of 6 and 12, you need about 9-12 hours of sleep each night. Teenagers typically need less sleep, about 8-10 hours, as outlined in Table 4.1. But everyone has their own unique, internal clock, telling them how much sleep they need.

TABLE 4.1: HOW MUCH EXERCISE AND SLEEP?

WHAT	HOW MUCH	TYPE	HOW IT CHANGES
SLEEP	IF YOU'RE BETWEEN 6-12 YEARS OLD YOU NEED 9-12 HOURS	YOU NEED BOTH REM AND NON-REM TYPE OF SLEEP.	YOUR SLEEP CYCLE SHIFTS AROUND AGE 12, WHEN THE BODY GETS TIRED LATER AT NIGHT.
	IF YOU'RE BETWEEN 13-18 YEARS OLD YOU NEED 8-10 HOURS		

WHAT	HOW MUCH	TYPE	HOW IT CHANGES
PHYSICAL ACTIVITY	YOU NEED ROUGHLY ONE HOUR MOST DAYS	ALL TYPES OF EXERCISE ARE GOOD: RUNNING, WALKING, BIKING, HIKING. BUT ALSO INCLUDE BONE BUILDING EXERCISES LIKE JUMPING; AND MUSCLE BUILDING EXERCISES LIKE PUSH-UPS AND SIT-UPS.	YOU MAY FIND THE DEMANDS OF SCHOOL, EXTRACURRICULAR ACTIVITIES, AND TECHNOLOGY RESULT IN LESS EXERCISE OR NATURAL WAYS TO BE ACTIVE.

BODY TALK: HOW TO GET TO SUPER FOCUS

So now that you know about why sleep and exercise are important, it's time to learn how to turn them into superpowers! Listen carefully and heed the messages about sleep and exercise, and everything in your life should come into focus.

YOUR BODY CLOCK

Did you know your body has a clock that talks to you about sleep? It's your circadian rhythm mentioned earlier. Circadian means to occur in a 24-hour cycle. The job of your body clock is tell you when to go to sleep and wake up, the same way that hunger and fullness tell you when and how much to eat and when to stop.

Your body clock communicates with you by sending signals of

tiredness such as yawning and heavy eyes. When you ignore these signals (or can't respond to them because of a sleepover or sickness), you'll find that you are tired at the wrong times, like the next day in math class or right before dinner. You're also more likely to be in a bad mood.

When you follow your internal clock's lead, you're rewarded by feeling well rested. Your body gives you positive signs like making it easier to fall asleep and wake up. During the day you feel more alert, in a good mood, and not so tired at random times.

What helps you use this superpower is having a sleep routine. This is doing the same set of activities, around the same time, most nights before bed. You want to choose relaxing activities like taking a bath, dimming the lights, and reading an enjoyable book (not a scary one!). Avoid doing things that get you excited like exercise, going on devices, staring at bright lights, and solving problems. If your worried thoughts overwhelm you, try keeping a notebook by your bed and writing them down so you can deal with them tomorrow. Sleep will actually help you come up with solutions!

When should it start? If you notice you get tired at 9:30, for instance, start your sleep routine an hour before that. Make getting ready for school the next day part of your routine as shown in Table 4.2. You will be amazed how a sleep routine helps you stay in touch with your body clock. Of course, you may not be able to do this every night and there will be times you stay up late. But when you are well rested most of the time, you'll bounce back quickly.

TABLE 4.2: THE BENEFITS OF A SLEEP ROUTINE

SLEEP ROUTINE	NO SLEEP ROUTINE

AN HOUR BEFORE YOUR BEDTIME, YOU TURN OFF YOUR DEVICES AND GET EVERYTHING READY FOR THE NEXT DAY.	YOU DO NOT WATCH THE CLOCK, CONTINUE TO STAY ON A DEVICE, DO YOUR HOMEWORK LATE, AND FAIL TO GET EVERYTHING READY.
START YOUR RELAXING ACTIVITIES IN THE SAME ORDER SUCH AS BATH, PJS AND BOOK.	YOU KEEP DOING ACTIVITIES/HOMEWORK AND TEXTING FRIENDS.
WHEN YOU FEEL TIRED AND READY FOR SLEEP, TURN LIGHTS OFF AND GO TO SLEEP.	YOU FINALLY GET TO BED AND THEN IT TAKES OVER AN HOUR TO FALL ASLEEP!
YOU WAKE UP FEELING RESTED, GET READY QUICKLY, AND ARE IN A GOOD MOOD.	IT'S HARD TO WAKE UP, STRESSFUL GETTING READY, AND YOU'RE IN A BAD MOOD.

FINICKY ACTIVITY SIGNALS

Using your physical activity powers is not at all like sleep or hunger. Your body doesn't talk to you by giving you a jolt of energy to tell you it's time to be active. It's actually the opposite. When you need activity, you usually are feeling low on energy. Consider how you feel after sitting on the couch all morning. You want to sit on the couch even more, right?

It actually takes movement to give you energy. This movement shifts the body to feel energetic. That's because it releases something called *endorphins*, natural chemicals in the brain that make you feel great. That's why if you're in a bad mood, simply going for a walk or bike ride can help you feel better.

Making activity enjoyable is very important. When you do

something you hate, your body doesn't get as much out of it. Plus, the more you like it, the more you'll want to do it. So it's okay to drop out of sports if that's not your thing. Just remember to replace it with something else.

The key with moving your body is to do it on a regular basis, not just during soccer season, while taking a dance class, or when you're in school. Because activity adds so much to your life, you'll want to keep doing it to be at your best. See Table 4.3 for some ideas.

TABLE 4.3: TYPES OF ACTIVITIES

TYPE	ACTIVITIES
AEROBIC (GETS HEART PUMPING)	NATURE WALKS, TREE CLIMBING, ROLLER-SKATING, BIKING, HIKING, JOGGING, RUNNING, DANCING, SPORTS GAMES LIKE SOCCER, TENNIS, TAG, SWIMMING, JUMPING ON A TRAMPOLINE, ZUMBA
BONE BUILDING (THERE'S IMPACT SO YOUR BONES GET STRONGER)	JUMPING ROPE, HOPPING, STAIR CLIMBING, TENNIS, DANCING, HIKING, AEROBICS
MUSCLE STRENGTHENING (USES MUSCLES)	EXERCISES THAT USE YOUR OWN BODY WEIGHT LIKE CARTWHEELS, PUSH-UPS/SIT-UPS, PLANKS, BENCH STEP-UPS, YOGA

Once you recognize how great exercise feels, you can set up an activity routine. Maybe during homework you take breaks and jump on a trampoline or even do jumping jacks. Or when you get home from school, you are active before homework and snack. Did you know activity breaks have been shown to stimulate the brain, making it easier to learn when you return? You can start "active" family traditions like riding your bike or hiking Saturday mornings.

Of course, you'll have rest days where you get little activity. Listen closely to your body to sense when you need a day to do nothing. This might be after a really active week or recovering from illness. Maybe you start some activity, but realize you just need to chill. Just listen to your body—it holds all the answers!

SUPER ADVICE!

When I was going through puberty, what I wish I would have known is that moving my body is good and healthy. I was a bookworm, so I was often at home reading or doing homework. My parents were always working, so they didn't encourage me to go out. Instead, I was always at home...And because of that, I developed a fear of movement and exercise. What I know now is that exercise can be very fulfilling and good for the soul. I know that not all of it is something that I enjoy. But, for instance, I love to dance. I wish my parents would have encouraged this interest when I was younger.

— Irina Gonzalez, freelance writer, editor,
and Latina journalist

BESTIES FOR FOCUS

Listening to and heeding your body's messages about sleep and activity gives you an advantage. With regular activity your brain is primed for learning and in a positive mood. Then when you sleep your body does important work for growth and memory. Everything you learned that day gets stored in your long-term memory so you're clear to start over the next day.

Together they work to keep you Super Focused every day. Like any true besties, they complement each other. And when one goes out of whack, the other can't function as well. You start staying up late and you're too tried for exercise. Stop exercising and your sleep isn't as deep.

Maybe for years a parent, friend, or teacher has been trying to get you to sleep more and be active. The key is to see how sleep and exercise make *your* life better. Always do it for *you*; not for anyone else.

These are how superpowers work; we need to experience them to believe them!

TIME TRAVEL

You don't need to Time Travel very far ahead to help you master Super Focus. When you're tempted to stay up late to study, take yourself to the next morning when you have to get up. How will you feel during the day in class? When you feel low on energy, imagine how you'll feel after moving your body. Just get started and see. Time Travel helps you see all the ways exercise and sleep will help you do everything better.

SUPER DECISIONS: SUPER FOCUS IN ACTION

Life doesn't always make it easy to honor your body with sleep and physical activity. Here are some examples of how to make Super Decisions.

LABELING YOURSELF: "NOT ACTIVE"

Sarah was never into sports much and she dreaded PE class. She played soccer until last year, mainly to please her parents. Now she is 12 and has a lot of homework and stays late at school for band practice. School and band are important to her so when she gets home, she does her homework and practices her instrument. Any free time is spent on her tablet and reading, and she feels tired and doesn't do much. Her interest in school also means she stays up late doing extra work. She tells herself she's just not an "active person," and gets very little exercise.

Super Knowledge helps Sarah realize that everyone is an active person—we were born to move. The key is finding activities she enjoys since not everyone is into sports and PE class. Sarah trades in some time on her tablet for riding her bike. Instead of late night studying, she starts doing a sleep routine. When she finds herself back to her old ways, she uses Time Travel to get back on track. Sarah is better able to focus, which translates to faster learning in band, better mood overall, and better grades, even when spending less time on homework.

Lack of Sleep

Jane plays soccer. She is on a year-round team but also has a big workload at school. Jane has two-hour practices three times a week. She rushes home and eats quickly, only to start doing homework and studying. Most nights she's up late, going between homework and surfing the internet. Her performance both in soccer and school begins to suffer. She is also easily irritable and finds herself crying at almost anything.

Jane's first thought is to get a tutor and soccer coach for help; but after learning about sleep, she decides to start there. With some help from her parents, she devises a plan to do homework more efficiently and without going online at all. For breaks, she jumps on the trampoline. On the days she doesn't have practice, she focuses on her homework and projects, and gets about an hour of relaxing time on her tablet. She starts a sleep routine and is now going to bed an hour earlier and sleeping more soundly. Jane improves both at school and at practice. She also feels better and doesn't get so easily upset over little things.

FROM PHYSICAL POWERS TO EMOTIONAL POWERS

Super Focus is about identifying your mind's exercise and sleep helpers and then putting them to work to sharpen your mind and life. This ends our Physical Powers section.

Mastering Super Focus along with your X-ray Vision, Appetite Signals, and Super Functioning makes you very powerful indeed. I hope you have a new appreciation for your growing and changing body. When you realize all it does for you and learn to take care of it, its superpowers will work magic in your lives.

But that's not all. You also need to learn about your Emotional Powers. Together with your Physical Powers, your life will be that much better. Let's start discovering!

PART 2

EMOTIONAL POWERS

"LIFE IS LOCOMOTION. IF YOU'RE NOT MOVING YOU'RE NOT LIVING. BUT THERE COMES A TIME WHEN YOU'VE GOT TO STOP RUNNING AWAY FROM THINGS AND YOU'VE GOT TO START RUNNING TOWARDS SOMETHING. YOU'VE GOT TO FORGE AHEAD. KEEP MOVING EVEN IF YOUR PATH ISN'T CLEAR. TRUST THAT YOU'LL FIND YOUR WAY."

- THE FLASH

CHAPTER 5

INTERNAL COMPASS

YOUR FEELINGS ARE YOUR BODY'S WAY OF SENDING YOU IMPORTANT information. It may be a bit whacky during puberty but by learning its language, you will experience a far more comfortable and satisfying life—and one that is more manageable. But before you can use your feelings as a compass, you need to know how the changes of puberty stir the pot of feelings.

SUPER KNOWLEDGE: THE STORM OF FEELINGS

Puberty can feel like a storm of emotions. But that's okay. Let's get at why you're experiencing emotions more intensely than before.

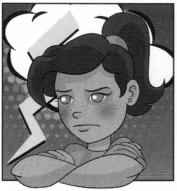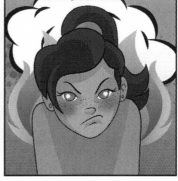

THE LOPSIDED BRAIN

During puberty, there's a lot going on in your brain that you need to know about. That's because the same hormones that instruct your body changes also cause changes in the big boss of your nervous system: your brain.

By age 5, your brain reaches 90% of adult size. So by the time puberty comes, the brain doesn't grow much more in size; but it does change on the inside. Many of these changes will affect how you feel.

Your brain experiences a gradual increase in white matter, called myelin. This speeds up communication so your brain works faster. One part of the brain is responsible for emotional responses (reacts by becoming angry or upset — "Things are never going to get better."), while another part is the voice of reason (tells you everything is going to be okay — "We'll find a solution.")

Here's the sticky part. The changes you experience occur first in your brain's emotional center–the *limbic system*. And this can make you feel. . . well, emotional. When you get upset, for instance, it can take a while to calm down. Feelings of sadness may feel overwhelming. You will also feel great feelings of joy and excitement. It's like a rollercoaster!

Because changes to the reasoning part of the brain (called the *prefrontal cortex)* lag behind the emotional part, it can feel lopsided. In other words, you're going to feel more emotional, and that's to be expected. Just imagine how boring it would be if tweens and teens developed reasoning first. You'd be like your parents! See Table 5.1 for more on these two parts of the brain.

TABLE 5.1: TWO PARTS OF THE BRAIN

EMOTIONAL CENTER (LIMBIC SYSTEM)	REASONING CENTER (PREFRONTAL CORTEX)
YOUR EMOTIONAL RESPONSES SUCH AS JOY, FEAR, ANGER, AND SADNESS	YOU CAN APPROPRIATELY RESPOND TO THE RANGE OF EMOTIONS AND CONTROL IMPULSES
YOU DESIRE TO DO OR HAVE SOMETHING NOW!	YOU CAN DELAY GRATIFICATION FOR A LONG-TERM GOAL (GIVE UP WHAT YOU WANT NOW FOR SOMETHING BETTER LATER)
YOU SEEK LEARNING ABOUT NOVEL AND NEW INFORMATION	YOU CAN TAKE WHAT YOU LEARN TO FORM STRATEGIES, PLAN, AND WORK TOWARDS A GOAL

A MIND FOR MOODINESS

There are your brain's emotional changes and then there's mood. While the two are related, it's worth noting the differences. It is thought that mood is affected more by the presence of estrogen, the hormone that causes your body to change during puberty. At the start of puberty, estrogen gradually increases in your body. Because you are being exposed to this hormone for the first time, it can affect your moods.

Mood is defined as "a prevailing attitude." Instead of a feeling that comes and goes, mood can be more constant. Think of it as the lens in which you see the world. When you are in a bad mood, everything seems bad. When you are in a good mood, everything seems wonderful.

Moodiness means your moods flip flop. And they can change in response to something—or for no reason at all. For example, maybe you find you're snapping at your sibling more than usual because you are stressed at school. Or you wake up one day in a really good mood but can find no reason why. The same is true for when things turn sour; there isn't always an explanation.

Another impact on your mood is being more self-conscious. This is feeling like everyone is watching and judging you, even when they aren't. This is the emotional part of the brain at work, worrying that you're doing everything wrong, or feeling awesome when things go your way.

For example, maybe you get in a bad mood because your teacher snaps at the class. Or your mood goes south because a friend doesn't wave hello. But in reality, your teacher is worried about her sick dog and your friend isn't mad at you, she just found out she bombed a test.

Your moods are changing and that's okay. As you will soon learn, there are lots of things you can learn from them!

WHAT IS PREMENSTRUAL SYNDROME (PMS)?

Once you get your cycles, the hormone estrogen will fluctuate along with your period. Estrogen levels increase until about a week before your period, when they decrease. This can result in moodiness along with other symptoms like pimples, bloating, feeling tired, headaches, and food cravings. This is called premenstrual syndrome (PMS) because it typically comes right before getting your period. There's good news, however. Mastering your physical powers can decrease the symptoms of PMS.

THE STRESS CONNECTION

Another side effect of puberty-related brain changes is how easily you can feel overstressed. Don't get me wrong, the brain needs stress to grow, change, and learn. But during puberty you are more sensitive to normal stress changing more quickly to overstressed mode.

Stress uses up energy in your brain. When it takes more energy than the brain has, you feel overwhelmed. High periods of stress once in awhile is not a problem; but feeling overstressed *all* the time can take a toll. That's because your body reacts by releasing stress hormones that cause your body to be ready to "fight or flight." So your body reacts like there's a threat, and your heart might pound faster and your breathing gets shallow.

It's important to know everyone reacts to stress differently. A stressor is an activity or situation that takes up more than the usual amount of energy. For example, even though *introverts* do like to be around people, extended periods of socializing can zap them of energy. *Extroverts* actually gain energy being around people, and too much time alone depletes them of energy. You may notice one friend gets stressed with school projects, while another just sails through. Everyone is so different.

The people in your life may not always understand your stressors because they don't get stressed about the same things. That's okay; just note the stressors in your life and we'll come back to this. Table 5.2 shows the difference between normal stress and overstress.

TABLE 5.2: THE DIFFERENT TYPES OF STRESS

HEALTHY STRESS	YOU GO ABOUT YOUR BUSINESS OF SCHOOL, FRIENDS, AND LIFE. YOU FEEL CONFIDENT THAT WITH SUPPORT YOU CAN GET EVERYTHING DONE.
STRESSOR	SITUATIONS OR EVENTS THAT TAKE UP EXTRA ENERGY. TOO MANY OF THESE TOGETHER CAN LEAD TO "OVERSTRESS."
OVERSTRESS	ENERGY DEPLETION LEADS TO FEELING OVER-WHELMED, DIFFICULTY CONCENTRATING, AND NOT FEELING LIKE YOURSELF.

BODY TALK: USING YOUR INTERNAL COMPASS

Now that you know what's going on inside you, it's time to learn how to respond. Think of feelings as your Internal Compass, telling you where to go. And you are about to learn the three very important steps to using this superpower!

1. LABEL FEELINGS

Your body talks to you through physical sensations. Before a test you might get a tight feeling in your chest or stomach. Tripping over something in front of people might make your face get red (called blushing). Some of these feelings are pleasant, like smiling when feeling joyful, and others are unpleasant, like blushing. Just remember, every feeling is there to tell you something important.

It's human nature to want to run from unpleasant feelings assuming something's wrong. It's also normal to want to do something to avoid them. But neither works, because the feelings stay inside you and will try to come out in other ways. Plus, you don't learn about what the feeling is trying to tell you. That's why the first step in using your Internal Compass is labeling your feelings.

When you have a feeling, sit with it and try to figure out what it is. If your family decides to cancel a weekend away because something else came up, you might feel like crying. That is disappointment. If you're unhappy with a new rule at home you weren't asked about, you might feel yourself getting worked up because it isn't fair. That is anger. You might feel a pit in your stomach every time you think about starting at a new school. That is fear or anxiety.

Your moods are related to emotions too. But you can't always find an exact reason for your mood—you're just in a bad (or good) mood! It's really important to accept how you are feeling, and not fight it. Label your mood like you do a feeling. When overstress occurs, your body sends strong messages. Some people get a stomachache or have diarrhea. Others feel on edge, like they can't relax because there's so much to do. It's hard to focus on tasks and sleep.

It's pretty amazing, actually. Your body talks to you through feelings. Your job is to figure out what those feelings mean. Look at the list in Table 5.3 and get in the habit of labeling your different feelings by putting a name (emotion) to it. Remember, emotions are neutral, so don't judge, but be curious about them.

TABLE 5.3: LABELING YOUR FEELINGS

SITUATION	FEELING	EMOTION
"THERE'S SO MUCH TO DO AT SCHOOL AND THE WORKLOAD IS INCREASING."	TIGHTNESS IN CHEST, MIND FEELS DISTRACTED, CAN'T RELAX	ANXIETY/ OVERSTRESSED
"NOTHING'S GOING MY WAY MY BEST FRIEND IS PULLING AWAY, I BOMBED A TEST, AND I DIDN'T GET ONE GOAL AT MY LAST SOCCER GAME."	FEEL LIKE CRYING, WISH THINGS COULD BE DIFFERENT	DISAPPOINT- MENT
"I CAN'T BELIEVE WE'RE MOVING. I'M GOING TO MISS MY FRIENDS SO MUCH."	SINKING FEELING IN YOUR STOMACH OR CHEST, LACK OF MOTIVATION, NOT ENJOYING USUAL ACTIVITIES	SADNESS

"THE TEACHER ALWAYS YELLS AT ME AND I DON'T LIKE IT."	FEEL HEAT RISE UP IN YOUR BODY MAKING YOU MAD	ANGER
"I FAILED TO KEEP A SECRET I PROMISED MY FRIEND I WOULD KEEP."	FEEL REGRET, WISHING YOU COULD CHANGE WHAT YOU DID	GUILT
"MY OLD FRIENDS FROM ELEMENTARY SCHOOL HAVE MOVED ON AND I DON'T HAVE NEW FRIENDS YET."	FEEL A LONGING FOR THE CONNEC- TION AND COMPANY OF OTHERS	LONELY
"HOW COME SHE GOT THE LEAD IN THE PLAY, I WORKED SO HARD ON IT. I WISH I WAS HER."	FEEL BAD OR DOWN ON YOURSELF	ENVY
"I TOLD A GROUP OF GIRLS WHO MY CRUSH IS AND NOW I REGRET IT."	RED FACE (BLUSH- ING), FEEL LIKE EVERYONE IS WATCHING AND WISH YOU COULD DISAP- PEAR	EMBARRASSED
"I DON'T KNOW THE RIGHT DECISION TO MAKE."	GOING BACK AND FORTH BETWEEN FEELING SURE AND NOT KNOWING	UNCERTAINTY

2. DISCOVER WHAT IT'S TRYING TO TELL YOU

Once you have labeled the feeling, try to figure out what the corresponding emotion is telling you. Some emotions just need to run their course like sadness—especially grief, like when you lose a beloved pet. Crying releases physical tension and may help you get over a loss, as can sharing your hurt feelings with a friend or family member. When you let difficult feelings pass through you, you feel better later and are able to move on.

Oftentimes difficult feelings are trying to tell you it's time to solve a problem. For example, maybe you feel overwhelmed every morning getting ready for school. The answer can be as simple as getting everything ready the night before school or doing homework earlier in the day to get to bed earlier. When overstress occurs the body is yelling: *Do something, I'm struggling!* When you get these signs take a timeout and consider what is contributing to it. Once you pinpoint your stressors, find ways to manage them. For example, you can't remove school projects and deadlines, but you can become more organized about doing them. Clutter in your room can be solved by cleaning it frequently. A friend disappointing you constantly may mean it's time to rethink the friendship.

Other emotions tell us it's time to grow and change. In these situations, you'll often need to communicate your needs to others. If you no longer enjoy an activity and start to dread it, you'll need to talk to your parents about it. If you're struggling with a certain subject, you'll want to let your teacher and parents know. If you're unhappy about something at home, you'll need to talk to family members. It's okay to make your needs known, and the adults in your life will appreciate it!

> It's also okay to have mixed/conflicting feelings. Many kids think that having uncertainty is wrong. It's best to be curious about your opposing wants and know it's healthy to have mixed feelings at times. You may need more information or time to sort out what you're feeling.

Pleasant emotions are trying to tell you something too. When you get excited by a subject or activity in school, it may mean it's time to explore it more. If you feel like your best self around a new friend, that signals you'll want to spend more time with that person. When you feel upbeat, note what contributes to that and try to do more of it. Just remember, your body is always communicating with you. It's not good nor bad, it's just communication.

Sometimes our thoughts are not in line with reality, causing unnecessary pain. This happens most frequently with worry and sadness. For example, you may worry all the time that you won't get a perfect grade on school projects. But is it realistic to set yourself up for perfection? After all, no one is perfect. Humans aren't meant to be. Or you may feel down because you get the feeling no one likes you, even though you have friends and a caring family. It's okay to question your thoughts because they are not facts. Sometimes your mind just needs more information.

If you have trouble shaking worry or sadness, there may be biological, genetic reasons and there are professionals that can help you. Be sure once again to make your needs known and talk to you parents or a trusted adult. Table 5.4 will help you figure out what different emotions are trying to tell you.

TABLE 5.4: EMOTION TALK & ACTION

WHAT IS THE EMOTION TRYING TO TELL ME?	WHAT TO DO
I NEED TO FEEL IT AND LET IT PASS	I NEED TO FEEL THIS EMOTION AND GET IT OUT OF ME. IT SHOWS ME WHAT IS IMPORTANT AND THAT I LOVE AND CARE ABOUT PEOPLE. I CAN LEAN ON SOMEONE FOR SUPPORT.

I NEED TO MAKE A CHANGE OR PROBLEM SOLVE	SOMETHING ISN'T WORKING FOR ME. I CAN BRAINSTORM IDEAS OR HAVE A FRIEND OR FAMILY MEMBER HELP ME.
I NEED TO CHECK IN WITH MY THOUGHTS	ASK YOURSELF: ARE THESE THOUGHTS TRUE OR IS THERE A BETTER WAY TO LOOK AT THIS SITUATION? DOES MY MIND HAVE ALL THE INFORMATION?

3. EXERCISE YOUR MIND

The key to your Internal Compass is discovering and taking action, but there's more you can do to bolster this superpower. Just the same way you exercise to make your body stronger, you can exercise to make your mind sharper. And you can use the SHARP method to get a regular practice going.

First is **S**, start with *mindfulness*. This is being aware of thoughts by paying close attention and reflecting on them. Often, daily thoughts are about things that haven't happened yet or stuff that has already occurred. It's easy to get stuck in your head thinking all day, instead of living your life. When you catch yourself thinking, make a mental note of it (or even write it down) and switch your focus back to what's going on right now. This is called being present.

Next is **H**, have a grateful attitude. Do you focus on problems all the time, or on what you don't have, instead of being grateful for what you do have? Don't worry, it's human nature to focus on problems. But with some conscious effort, you can catch yourself and develop a grateful attitude. School can be a pain, but aren't you lucky to get an education? Got a difficult teacher? Be grateful for what that teacher is teaching you. Maybe you are learning patience and compassion, which will make you stronger.

Next is **A, a**lways be kind to yourself, referred to as *self-compassion*. When you are hard on yourself for not doing great on that test or saying the wrong thing, it creates even more stress. Plus, it decreases your motivation to take action and problem solve. Everyone makes mistakes and feels stress about life, even your mom and dad. Talk to yourself like you would to a friend and you'll find you bounce back quicker.

Next is **R, r**edirect to energy-giving activities. These are activities that help you manage stress like taking a bath, walking, deep breathing, reading a book, talking to friends or family, drawing, jumping, getting enough sleep, and exercising. It's natural to want to escape stress by blaming someone else for it, eating when not hungry, excessively playing video games or binge watching TV. Even though these activities take your mind off stress, they deplete your energy. And when you're done, the stressor seems worse than before.

Last is **P, p**ause before making decisions. When you're in the middle of an emotion, like fear or anger, you have trouble accessing the reasoning part of the brain. In other words, the door that connects the emotional and reasoning brain is shut. Instead of making a decision right then and there, find an activity that helps you calm down or simply take some deep breaths. Getting back to calm will open the door to your reasoning brain, which helps you make a better decision.

The key with each of these is practice. In Table 5.5, you can get ideas for daily activities that are simple to do. You will be amazed at how they transform your mood and make you realize that you can handle anything.

TABLE 5.5: SHARP PRACTICE

SHARP ACRONYM	HOW IT HELPS	PRACTICE
START WITH MINDFULNESS	ENJOY YOUR LIFE MORE!	SIT IN SILENCE FOR 5 MINUTES A DAY AND FOCUS ON YOUR BREATHING. WHEN THOUGHTS COME UP, MAKE A NOTE AND GO BACK TO FOCUSING ON YOUR BREATHING.
HAVE A GRATEFUL ATTITUDE	BETTER MOODS MORE OFTEN!	KEEP A JOURNAL AND WRITE THREE THINGS YOU ARE GRATEFUL FOR EVERY DAY.
ALWAYS BE KIND TO YOURSELF	LESS STRESS AND WORRY!	WHEN YOU ARE HARD ON YOURSELF, WRITE IN YOUR JOURNAL. HOW CAN YOU BE KINDER TO YOURSELF? REMEMBER THAT EVERY HUMAN FEELS THESE FEELINGS FROM TIME TO TIME.
REDIRECT TO ENERGY GIVING ACTIVITIES	STRESS FEELS MANAGEABLE!	WHEN FEELING STRESSED, FIRST CHECK TO SEE IF YOU ARE GETTING ENOUGH SLEEP, ACTIVITY, AND EATING NUTRITIOUS FOODS. KEEP A LIST OF ACTIVITIES THAT GIVE YOU ENERGY AND GO TO THAT LIST FOR A BREAK.

PAUSE BEFORE MAKING DECISIONS	BETTER DECISIONS!	REGULARLY PRACTICE DEEP BREATHING BY TAKING A DEEP BREATH IN THROUGH YOUR NOSE, HOLD YOUR BREATH FOR A FEW SECONDS, AND THEN BREATHE OUT THROUGH YOUR MOUTH. THIS SENDS A MESSAGE TO YOUR BODY THAT IT'S OKAY FOR IT TO CALM DOWN.

TIME TRAVEL!

It's not always easy working through difficult feelings. But if you choose not to, time traveling shows you all the ways your feelings stay with you. So imagine yourself in a month from now if you don't tell your parents you no longer enjoy a sport. You can see you have to drag yourself to practice and it turns your mood sour. Talking to them now may be unpleasant, but it will bring you closer to a solution. Maybe you don't understand your math homework. By avoiding dealing with the emotion of uncertainty, you'll have to stay up late finishing it night after night. Although it takes effort to tell your teacher and parents your struggle, they can give you the support you need to get over the problem. The other side to difficult feelings is problem solving and relief.

SUPER ADVICE

There are amazing upsides to adolescence, just like there are fabulous upsides to childhood and adulthood. During adolescence, you will stretch and grow physically, but also emotionally. Both can hurt a little, and can be exhilarating and exhausting. All of it will teach you things that you'll use for the rest of your life. Make it all count. Sisters: live big, love yourself, and be kind to others.

—Marnie Goldenberg, Sex Education Specialist

SUPER DECISIONS: INTERNAL COMPASS IN ACTION

Here are examples of how to use your Internal Compass to get through life's struggles.

BAD MOOD ZEUS

Tina had many tough mornings. She'd wake up late, figure out something to wear, and skip breakfast. She'd get to school on time but soon found herself hungry and crabby. Many days she realized she forgot something she needed to turn in. She was in a bad mood most of the time and just figured she didn't like school. She couldn't wait for the day to be over.

Super Knowledge helped Tina realize this was her body's way of telling her something—it's time for a change. Like many people do, she was mistaking her Internal Compass for the fact that something was wrong. Time Travel showed her that school was only going to get more difficult and she needed to figure things out now.

So Tina noticed what she was feeling. Her running around in the morning was causing overstress, leading her to feel overwhelmed. After talking to her mom, they decided she'd put her clothes out the night before and create a checklist for what needs to go in her backpack. They also brainstormed quick breakfast ideas that she could grab and go, since her school starts early. To help her moods, Tina started a gratitude journal and wrote three things she was grateful for every day, with one being school related.

After a week of this new routine, Tina was enjoying school more and in a better mood. She still had bad mood days but learned how to handle them.

SCHOOL STRESS

Robin did well at school and was a straight-A student. Her teachers loved her and everyone came to her for questions when they didn't understand something. Her parents praised her for her accomplishments and Robin liked that. But Robin had been noticing she felt pressure to be "perfect" at school. She worried that if her grades fell or she didn't do well at soccer, she'd disappoint everyone. She started having stomachaches and found that her worry kept her awake at night.

When Robin labeled her feelings she discovered the emotion she's having is anxiety. As tough as it was, she confided in her mom about it. Her mom could hardly believe it, and thanked her for coming to her. Together they figured out Robin's thinking that she had to be perfect was putting too much pressure on her. She learned that while her parents wanted her to do well, they especially wanted her to be happy. Mistakes were okay!

Knowing this gave Robin's mind the information it needed and she felt better instantly. She started to be kinder to herself and realized that no one is perfect; and she was no exception. She still did well in school and soccer but enjoyed them even more because she stopped feeling so much pressure to be perfect. Her stomachaches went away and she started to sleep better.

FROM INTERNAL COMPASS TO SUPER FRIENDS

Internal Compass is discovering how your mind is developing and using your feelings and emotions to problem solve and live a better life. Be sure to ask a trusted adult to help you with what you are feeling.

Next, the importance of being a Super Friend and choosing other Super Friends to hang out with.

CHAPTER 6

SUPER FRIENDS

YOUR WORLD IS OPENING UP. AND PART OF THIS MEANS SCHOOL and friends feel more important than ever. Here's a secret: bodies feel great when they are connected to others, and not so great when they feel lonely. The key is to find your Super Friends, the people that support you and want you to be happy.

SUPER KNOWLEDGE: A MIND MADE FOR CONNECTION

As friends take center stage during this time in your life, there's lots you need to know. Let's start with why you want to fit in so badly.

FITTING IN OR BELONGING?

The human brain is wired for connection, and meaningful relationships are important for lifelong health. Strong relationships decrease the amount of stress hormones that run through your body. The changes in your brain during puberty sensitize you to your social world. That means you will be (or are) more focused on friendships and their importance in your life.

We tend to think of learning in terms of school work, but this is also a time of social learning. You are learning about the kind of friends you want in your life and the kind of friend you want to be. You are learning how to handle difficult situations that involve others. You are learning how to treat others, stand up for yourself or a friend, and how not to lose your true self in friendships. Like any type of learning, there will be ups and downs.

Because your brain is preparing you for the social world, it's normal to want to fit in. You might experiment with what your friends are doing when it comes to music, food, and clothes. This can help because it exposes you to new things. It can become a problem when you feel you *have* to act a certain way to keep a friend.

What makes you feel connected to others isn't fitting in; it's feeling like you belong. That means you feel valued and loved for who you are. Super Friends accept you as you are, can be trusted, and want you to be happy. On the other hand, friends that make you feel like you need to act a certain way to be accepted or put you down, are not true friends. Table 6.1 lists what makes a Super Friend.

TABLE 6.1: WHAT MAKES A SUPER FRIEND?

FRIEND QUALITIES YOU WANT	FRIEND QUALITIES TO QUESTION
CAN BE YOURSELF	HAVE TO ACT A CERTAIN WAY TO BE HER FRIEND
TREATS YOU WELL	DOESN'T TREAT YOU WELL/IS INCONSIDERATE
DOESN'T PRESSURE YOU TO DO SOMETHING AFTER YOU SAID NO	KEEPS PRESSURING YOU TO DO SOMETHING AFTER YOU'VE MADE IT CLEAR YOU DON'T WANT TO

WELCOMES YOUR OTHER FRIENDS	IS THREATENED BY YOUR OTHER FRIENDS
CAN BE TRUSTED	NOT TRUSTWORTHY
IS RELIABLE MOST OF THE TIME	ALWAYS LETTING YOU DOWN
TREATS THE PEOPLE AROUND HER RESPECT-FULLY	TALKS BADLY ABOUT OTHERS
HAPPY FOR YOU WHEN YOU SUCCEED	LESSENS OR PUTS DOWN YOUR ACCOMPLISHMENTS
IS HONEST WITH THEM-SELVES AND YOU	ACTS DISHONESTLY
IS A GOOD LISTENER	MOSTLY TALKS ABOUT HERSELF

BULLY BASICS

Because during puberty the brain focuses on friends and fitting in, some kids are tempted to use power to rise to the top of the social ladder. When someone bullies, they use their power negatively towards someone, which includes repeated aggressive or mean-spirited behavior.

There are different types of bullying listed in Table 6.2. *Verbal bullying* uses words to make fun of or start rumors about someone. *Physical bullying* uses pushing, hitting, blocking, or unwanted physical contact to intimidate someone. *Relational bullying* uses tactics to purposely exclude people from a group, such as ignoring someone at the lunch table. Last is *cyber bullying* which is bullying that occurs online in the form of texts, tweets, and mean comments.

TABLE 6.2: TYPES OF BULLYING

TYPE OF BULLYING	WHAT IT IS	EXAMPLE
VERBAL	USING WORDS TO PUT SOMEONE DOWN	STARTING FALSE RUMORS ABOUT SOMEONE TO MAKE THEM SUFFER
PHYSICAL	USING PHYSICAL GESTURES TO TERRORIZE SOMEONE	BLOCKING SOMEONE EVERY DAY, KEEPING THEM FROM THE LUNCH ROOM
RELATIONAL	EXCLUDING OTHERS FROM A GROUP	DELIBERATELY LEAVING SOMEONE OUT OF A CONVERSATION THAT IS IN THE GROUP; NOT LOOKING AT THEM
CYBER BULLYING	BULLING OVER THE INTERNET	LEAVING MEAN COMMENTS OR OUTRIGHT LIES ABOUT SOMEONE ONLINE

The most common form of bullying among girls is relational bullying. This can happen when friends form groups, always hanging out with the same people. Forming groups is normal and not always bad, as we tend to become friends with people who share our interests. But there is a downside to that too, and this is where relational bullying can come in. Maybe the leader of the group purposely excludes other girls or doesn't allow their friends to have friends outside the group. Maybe they spread rumors about other girls or talk badly about them behind their backs.

Remember the last chapter when we talked about emotions? Kids who bully may simply be feeling bad themselves—dealing with difficult emotions—and end up bullying because they don't know what to do with their feelings. Their escape from emotions might be to feel important or popular at school. And when they make others feel less important, it boosts how they feel about themselves. Sometimes kids who bully are popular, but when they misuse power, they are usually sad inside. Just remember that if someone is bullying you, it usually has more to do with what is going on with them, than anything wrong with you. And you need to let your parents or a trusted adult know if it is happening to you so you can problem solve together.

SUPER ADVICE

Bullies and gossips are more insecure than their targets. "Haters" need your sympathy and prayers more than your hurt and anger.
— Xian Horn, is a joyful half-Asian woman with Cerebral Palsy, serving as writer, mentor, and positivity activist.

THE IMPORTANCE OF EMPATHY

Oftentimes, people that look or act different are more likely to be singled out and bullied. What's usually behind this is that people don't understand why that person is different. It's all too easy to fear what you don't understand. But something else important is missing, and that's considering what isn't different about that person: her feelings.

We are more alike than we are different. Yeah, we have different likes, dislikes, and characteristics, but we all feel the same range of emotions. And because the mind is wired for connection, nothing hurts more than being rejected or made to feel less of a person because of who you are. Being sent a message that you are flawed hurts very badly. The emotion most often attached to this feeling is shame.

Because this book is about growing a healthy body, you need to know that the most common reason kids get bullied is for their size. For example, heavy kids may get called fat, be made fun of, or excluded from groups. This only makes them feel worse about their body, making them less likely to take care of it.

The misunderstanding here is that people wrongly believe a person's size is 100% in their control. And you know from reading the first section this is not the case. Someone's size and shape is personal, just as other private matters are. It says absolutely nothing about who the person is.

The real key is to work on strengthening your empathy muscle. Empathy is putting yourself in someone else's shoes and considering how they feel. This doesn't mean you have to be friends with everyone. It only means that you treat everyone with respect. Like the golden rule says, "treat others the way you want to be treated."

GET COMFORTABLE WITH DIVERSITY

Get curious about all the ways people can act and look different from you. Ask your parents about volunteer opportunities to help those less fortunate and read books about how different people overcome adversity. Get to know other cultures through travel or documentaries. Also notice how people are the same inside. Most just want to be happy, feel loved, and spend time with family and friends. A world where everybody looks and acts the same would be boring!

BODY TALK: CONNECTING WITH OTHERS

Your body is talking to you all the time about your social world. Let's find out how to use this superpower to make Super Friends!

COMPARE WITH CAUTION

Comparing yourself to others is one way you learn about your social world. You may look at a friend and notice the ways in which she's different than you. Maybe she does better in math and sports or she doesn't have the same body shape as you. After comparing, your body sends messages that these comparisons are good, bad, or neutral. Knowing this is normal and how best to handle these comparisons is important.

Let's start with the good. You may find that there is an area in which you tend to do better than most people. It may be in a subject or activity, and it can give you a boost. A not so helpful reaction would be to tie "who you are" to this activity or skill. That could cause you stress to stay the best, and cause incredible disappointment when you make mistakes. Feeling superior to others isn't helpful, either.

A better way to handle ways in which you excel is to note your areas of talent. A talent is something you have a natural inclination towards. And when you add learning, passion, and practice to it, you gain a strength that can have a positive impact on the world. Stay humble with your talents and remember that they don't define you, but are simply an extension of you. Every person in the world has unique talents.

Sometimes when you compare yourself to others you feel bad. The brain naturally focuses on what it doesn't have. So if you want a pet and your friend has three, you may feel envious. If someone at your school gets lots of attention because they are outgoing, you might think something is wrong with you because you are more quiet.

The key is not to take envy too seriously, as we all feel it from time to time. In some cases, it's trying to tell you something. Maybe you feel envious of someone who loves basketball because you know you don't love soccer anymore and want to try something new. Or feeling jealous of your cousin's close friendships might be the motivation you need to branch out and make new friends. Table 6.3 helps you figure out the helpful and not so helpful ways to use social comparisons.

The worst thing you can do is let envy corrode your heart and life. Because you know what? Someone is looking at your life right now and feeling envious of you. No one's life is perfect, even though it can seem that way on the outside.

TABLE 6.3: SOCIAL COMPARISONS

HELPFUL	NOT SO HELPFUL
FIGURE OUT WHAT YOUR UNIQUE TALENTS ARE AND/OR WHAT YOU ENJOY DOING	THINK YOU ARE SUPERIOR OR DEFINED BY WHAT YOU DO
SEE IF THE ENVY YOU FEEL IS TRYING TO TELL YOU SOMETHING	LET ENVY MAKE YOU THINK YOUR LIFE WILL NEVER BE GOOD ENOUGH
REALIZE SOME ENVY IS NORMAL AND NOT TO BE TAKEN SO SERIOUSLY	TRY TO BE LIKE OTHERS YOU ENVY, EVEN THOUGH THAT ISN'T RIGHT FOR YOU

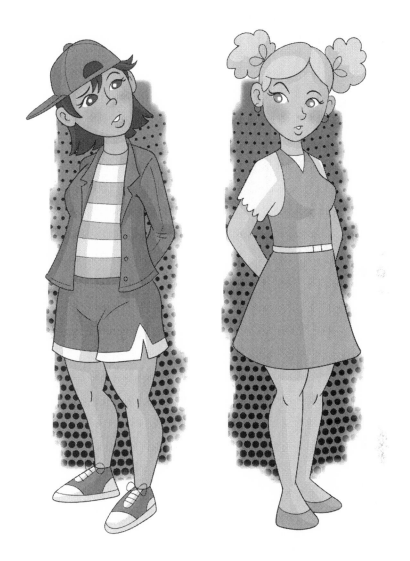

SUPER FRIEND FEELINGS

We already talked about qualities of a Super Friend, but how does your body talk to you about how this area of your life is going? In lots of ways.

Some signs a friendship is on the wrong track is how you feel before meeting up with someone. If you feel nervous you might say the wrong thing, maybe you don't feel like you can be yourself. If you're always disappointed by someone, she may not be reliable. If you feel you can't talk about what is going on with you, she may not be supportive or is too focused on herself.

If you're part of a group, consider how that group treats others. You may be treated well, but if they are always talking bad about others, you might feel guilty associating with them, even when you don't participate. But you might feel insecure because if they talk that bad about others, you might wonder if they do the same about you when you're not around. These feelings are helping you decide about friendships, so listen to them closely. And feel free to talk to someone about it too.

While nobody's perfect and even the best of friend will make mistakes, you want to feel confident about your friendships. That doesn't mean you have to cut off people at the first sign of trouble; but rather, use your feelings as a compass to help you find Super Friends. Sometimes girls your age go through tough times and unknowingly take it out on their friends. In time they can change and maybe a friendship can be reborn later.

On the flipside, when you get mostly positive feelings from friends, you know they are keepers. You can be yourself, you feel supported, and you like how they treat others. Table 6.4 can help you figure out your friend feelings.

TABLE 6.4: FRIEND FEELINGS

EMOTIONS	WATCH OUT	GOOD SIGN
EMBARRASSED	YOU CAN'T BE YOURSELF; YOU MIGHT FEEL EMBARRASSED ABOUT SAYING THE WRONG THING.	AROUND CLOSE FRIENDS YOU TEND TO FEEL LESS EMBARRASSED.
GUILTY	YOU FEEL GUILTY FOR TALKING ABOUT OTHERS OR DOING SOMETHING YOU DON'T WANT TO DO.	CLOSE FRIENDS ALLOW YOU TO SAY 'NO' AND TREAT OTHERS WELL.
LONELY	EVEN THOUGH YOU HANG OUT, YOU STILL FEEL LONELY.	WITH CLOSE FRIENDS YOU DON'T FEEL LONELY, YOU FEEL VALUED.
DISAPPOINTED	YOU ARE LET DOWN REPEATEDLY BY A FRIEND, WHICH CAN LEAD TO DISAPPOINT-MENT.	SOME DISAPPOINT-MENT IS NORMAL, BUT OVERALL YOU FEEL YOUR FRIEND IS SUPPORTIVE AND RELIABLE.
DRAINED	FRIEND ACTS LIKE A VICTIM/ALWAYS COMPLAINING AND BLAMING OTHERS. YOU'RE ALWAYS FOCUSED ON HER ISSUES.	YOUR FRIEND HAS PROBLEMS BUT TAKES RESPONSIBIL-ITY FOR THEM AND HAS TIME TO LISTEN TO WHAT'S BUGGING YOU.

COMMUNITY COUNTS

We can't touch on social connections without mentioning communities. A *community* is a group of people living, working, or doing a particular activity in the same area. For example, if you go to school you have a school community. If you are home-schooled, you likely have friends that are also homeschooled. You probably find you are a part of a variety of smaller communities, based on your interests. For example, church may be one and sports, another. Or if you like acting you can find a theater community in your area.

Being part of a community has health benefits just like friend-ships do. It's nice to know we are surrounded by people who care about our well-being and do, like, or believe, the same things we do. This can buffer the stress we feel, which helps our body.

One key benefit of a community is that a group of people can solve problems better than any one person can. If a challenge comes up, for instance, many people can get together to come up with potential solutions. When you go through challenges—or have difficulty making a big decision—you can tap into your communities for help. Lean on others when you don't feel so strong. And then you can be there for others when they need support.

If you don't feel part of a community, you can work toward creating one, be more active in communities you already belong to, or look for social settings that appeal to you. Many schools have clubs that exist or can be created. You'd be surprised how many other people share your interests. You won't know the possibilities until you try to connect with others.

TIME TRAVEL

Because our mind is made for connection, it can be tempting to hold on to friendships that aren't working. Time Travel shows you that if you do that, you'll miss out on the Super Friends you might have met along the way. So pulling away from a group may cause loneliness today, but it also opens you up to new friends and experiences in the future. And if you are caught up in envy of others, think how frustrated you'll feel trying to be something you're not. Embracing who you are now means you'll grow as a person and be happier in the future.

SUPER DECISIONS: SUPER FRIENDS IN ACTION

Here are examples of the power of finding and being a Super Friend.

THE INTROVERT

Diane was an introvert and often found herself envious of girls that were more outgoing, including her best friend. She thought how great it would be to be able to talk to anyone and be the life of the party. She felt bad about herself and sometimes wondered who would want to be her friend. Most of her life she was told, "You're so quiet," and she was letting it get her down.

After gaining Super Knowledge, she considered what this emotion was trying to tell her. She was making the mistake of thinking that envy meant something was wrong with her. She realized she needed to embrace who she is the same way her friends embrace who they are. Changing her personality was not a superpower she had, and Time Travel showed her that trying to be something she wasn't would make her miserable.

Because she really liked writing, she decided to join a writing club at school, which led to her trying out to be a reporter for the yearbook the following year. She also realized that being more introverted makes her an excellent listener—perfect for the journalistic reporting she ended up doing. She now understands that her friends appreciate her for who she is, and yes, that's on the quiet side. But that's okay!

FRIENDSHIP TROUBLE

Charlotte was new to middle school and she quickly formed a new group of friends. At first this was fun because she liked having the safety of a group in a new, bigger school. But after a while she noticed it just didn't feel right. When she went against what her group liked, they made sly comments that made her feel embarrassed. She often felt guilty when they all gossiped together about other girls. The leader of the group didn't like it when Charlotte sat with other girls. Even though she had these friends, Charlotte felt lonely.

With some Super Knowledge, Charlotte realized these feelings were telling her something, so she talked to her mom about it. She decided it was time to hang out with different people. Her old group didn't like it; and although she still sat with them at times and said hello, she decided having only one group of friends was limiting her. By the end of the year she had several groups she could sit with at lunch and had a few really close friends that she felt she could be herself around.

HIGH SCHOOL WOES

Jody was in 8th grade and had to make a decision about high school. She was an excellent softball player and considered a private school that excelled in sports. But the public school near her would be where most of her friends went. Her parents were supportive but left it up to Jody to decide.

Jody decided to tap into her community. She checked with her mom to see if she knew anyone currently playing softball at either school. By reaching out to friends, her mom found a few names. Jody met with them and asked questions. She also tapped into her school community of counselors and they gave her more information about both schools. After she talked to several people, she decided to attend the private school. She now feels confident with her decision instead of being unsure.

FROM SUPER FRIENDS TO SUPER YOU!

Super Friends means acknowledging the importance of connection and being thoughtful when forming and maintaining friendships.

Now it's time to focus on getting to know yourself and what excites you.

CHAPTER 7

SUPER YOU!

YOU ARE NOT ONLY LEARNING ABOUT YOUR GROWING BODY, CHANGING emotions, and social situations, you are learning about yourself and what makes you happy. Let's start with what you need to know about discovering your Super You during puberty and beyond.

SUPER KNOWLEDGE: THE HARD THING CAN BE THE RIGHT THING

It's not always easy discovering more about yourself, but it sure is worth it. Let's learn about the character traits you need to blossom.

WHY INDEPENDENCE?

Who doesn't like everything being done for them? Breakfast made, clothes clean and folded, and everything you need for the school project in your room ready to go. Problem is, when you reach double digits you are not only capable of doing more for yourself, but doing things for yourself makes you a stronger person.

Our *culture* puts a lot of emphasis on achievement and not enough on life skills. So it's not uncommon for someone to reach college age getting straight As, but does not know how to cook, do laundry, make decisions on her own, or complete a project without help. Even though it's never too late to learn these skills, it's better to learn now while your brain is changing.

When you don't build independence your brain jumps to the conclusion that you *can't* do things and builds up a resistance to trying them. This makes you feel less in control of your life. This can decrease confidence and keep you too reliant on others to get basic tasks done.

Building independence is an important part of adolescence. That doesn't mean you do everything yourself, but that you start learning how to do things for yourself. You can think of your parents as coaches. They can help you learn, but if they just do everything for you, that's not coaching. Coaches don't play the game for the kids. No, they have them practice and provide feedback until they get better. Table 7.1 summarizes easy steps to learning independent-minded skills.

TABLE 7.1: LEARNING STEPS

1. WATCH YOUR PARENTS DO IT	ASK YOUR PARENTS IF YOU CAN WATCH THEM DO SOMETHING AND EXPLAIN HOW THEY DO IT
2. DO IT TOGETHER	DO IT WITH THEM SEVERAL TIMES TIMES
3. HAVE THEM WATCH YOU DO IT AND PROVIDE FEEDBACK	WHEN YOU'RE READY, DO IT ON YOUR OWN AND ASK THEM TO GIVE YOU FEEDBACK UNTIL YOU ARE TOTALLY INDEPENDENT AT THE TASK.

TAP INTO YOUR VALUES AND CHARACTER

It's normal to ask the question....*who am I?* After all, you are gradually adopting your own unique identity, the kind of person you want to be. The good news is you have lots of time to figure it out. As you get older you're going to be confronted with making decisions that, over time, add up to the type of person you will become. It helps to consider your values and character.

Values are what you believe is most important in life. Of course, your parents heavily influence your values; but why not think about them yourself? Values can include specific beliefs about God and religion, family, health, friendship, learning, work, and play.

Character is more about how you live your values. Many of the women and men you study in history class had what is referred to as "strong character." They stood up for what they believed in, even when it was hard, and didn't give up. Their lives had meaning, which is why we like to share their stories and are amazed at how courageously they lived.

An organization called Character Counts! ® details 6 general pillars of character summarized in Table 7.2, but feel free to expand on this list. These include trustworthiness, respect, responsibility, fairness, caring, and citizenship. It's important to periodically check in to see if your values are lining up with your behavior. If there's a mismatch, it may be time to change something. For example, if someone values friendship but isn't trustworthy in her actions, that limits relationship building.

Character is not about perfection, which is setting unrealistic standards for yourself and feeling stressed about what others think. Quite the contrary, adopting a strong character is about learning from mistakes and acting honorably, even when no one is watching. Although this isn't always easy, it has many rewards, one of which is self-respect.

TABLE 7.2: CHARACTER EXAMPLES

THE 6 PILLARS OF CHARACTER*	EXAMPLES
TRUSTWORTHI-NESS	BE HONEST, DO WHAT YOU SAY YOU'RE GOING TO DO, STAND BY FAMILY AND FRIENDS, AND BE DEPENDABLE
RESPECT	TREAT OTHERS THE WAY YOU WANT TO BE TREATED, ACCEPT DIFFERENCES, USE GOOD MANNERS, AND HANDLE DISAGREEMENTS PEACEFULLY
RESPONSIBILITY	DON'T GIVE UP EASILY, PLAN AHEAD, UTILIZE SELF-DISCIPLINE, BE ACCOUNTABLE FOR YOUR ACTIONS, AND ADMIT MISTAKES
FAIRNESS	LISTEN AND BE OPEN MINDED, FOLLOW RULES, AND DON'T RUSH TO BLAME OTHERS
CARING	BE GRATEFUL, BE KIND TO OTHERS, HELP THOSE IN NEED, BE CHARITABLE, AND FORGIVE EASILY
CITIZENSHIP	GET INVOLVED IN YOUR SCHOOL AND/OR COMMUNITY, BE A GOOD NEIGHBOR, VOTE, VOLUNTEER, AND RESPECT AUTHORITY

*Used with permission by Michael Josephson, President & Founder of the Josephson Institute of Ethics

ADOPT A GROWTH MINDSET (WITH INSIDE GOALS)

As you learn and grow as a person, having a *growth mindset* is vital. A growth mindset is believing that you can get better at something with effort and practice. People are not born as successes or failures; they can learn and improve with doing virtually anything. While a growth mindset is usually discussed in regards to school and intelligence, it applies to everything from cleaning your room, to cooking, to public speaking.

A fixed mindset is believing that abilities and intelligence are fixed and can't be changed. So someone might say, "I'm not good at X," but if they wanted to, they could learn, practice, and get better. When people have a fixed mindset they are less likely to take on new challenges for fear they will fail. To them, not being able to do something means they are flawed. But this is not true!

Talent does play a role and has its place. You can think of talent as giving people a head start. Often, but not always, what people are talented in is also what they are passionate about. And this passion and desire makes them want to learn more and get better. But talent without learning and practice only gets you so far. Just remember, you don't have to have a special talent to learn how to do something.

It can be tough to have a growth mindset when you are focused on doing something to please teachers or parents. These "outside goals" are based on what others value and are more focused on outcomes. This is different from "inside goals" that come from what *you* value and are focused more on enjoying the process.

For example, in school you can focus on getting straight As (outside) or you can focus on learning and personal growth (inside). With friends you can focus on creating close, meaningful relationships (inside) or being popular (outside). When it comes to your body you can focus on building strong health (inside) or looking a certain way (outside).

Your growth is limited with a fixed mindset and outside goals. But when you adopt a growth mindset with inside goals, your growth and potential will skyrocket.

What do building character, a growth mindset, and inside goals have in common? How you view mistakes and setbacks. These aren't bad, or about disappointing others, but are ways to learn and get better. Sometimes it's not even a mistake—it's just realizing that what you are doing is no longer working. Everybody makes mistakes and has setbacks. Embrace them and use them as learning tools to help you grow.

SUPER ADVICE

The "oops" you have made are not mistakes or regrets per se; they are lessons to help you and/or others do better. It may even be a blessing in disguise. You may not see it now; it may take time to see what the lesson or blessing is. Be patient with yourself. Let your story unfold.

— Xian Horn, is a joyful half-Asian woman with Cerebral Palsy, serving as writer, mentor, and positivity activist

BODY TALK: FEELING PROUD

As you discover yourself, your body talks to you. Learning to read its signals is key to becoming Super You! Many adults would benefit from this too!

THE ULTIMATE REWARD

From an early age children are told to do the right thing to please an adult or get a tangible reward. We've already pointed out the problem with outside goals during adolescence. Now let's focus more on *why*, by considering how your body responds to what we'll call "Character Grows Inside."

How does your body talk to you about character? Well, how do you feel when you fall short on your standards, like telling a

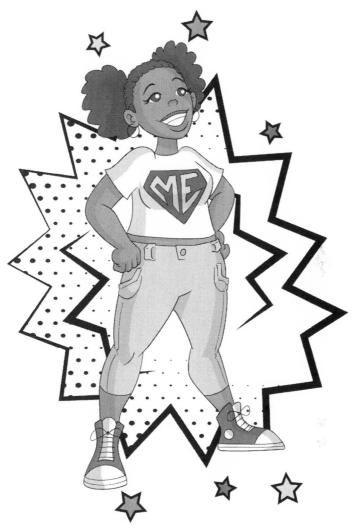

lie? You probably feel guilty, right? The lie may have helped in the short term, but then you end up feeling bad about yourself, even when no one finds out. Dropping out of an activity you committed to may get you out of the dreaded task, but following it through until it's done is the right thing to do. And who knows? By the end you may find you've changed your mind about the task—and feel better about yourself too!

The end result of being a person of strong character is not a reward or even praise from someone. It's that feeling of satisfaction inside that you did the right thing. It makes you happier, stronger, and you take pride in yourself.

Having a growth mindset and inside goals is very rewarding as well. With a growth mindset you feel challenged, are actively involved with life, and are learning new things. Your body responds to inside goals with feelings of satisfaction and meaning. Whether you get rewarded or not doesn't matter as much because you're fully involved in the experience. In other words, you're doing it to improve yourself, not to get that stamp of approval from others.

Ironically, a growth mindset and inside goals are more likely to lead to better outcomes, like good grades and better performance in sports. But that's not *why* you're doing it, which brings more satisfaction and happiness to your life.

On the other hand, what we'll call "Low Character Fixates Outside" is more stressful as detailed in Table 7.3. Knowing you are not living up to your standards (even when others don't know) means you're constantly disappointed in yourself. A fixed mindset usually results in feeling unchallenged, bored, and fearful of trying new things. And because outside goals are tied to others' approval, there is more stress involved, even when you are excelling.

TABLE 7.3: CHARACTER GROWS INSIDE

Life Factor	Feeling Fulfilled	Life Factor	Feeling Stressed
CHARACTER (STRONG)	HAVING A STRONG CHARACTER MAKES YOU FEEL PROUD AND GOOD ABOUT YOURSELF.	LOW CHARACTER	FALLING SHORT IN CHARACTER MAKES YOU FEEL BAD ABOUT YOURSELF EVEN THOUGH IT CAN MAKE LIFE EASIER IN THE SHORT TERM.
GROWS (GROWTH MINDSET)	A GROWTH MINDSET MAKES YOU A BETTER LEARNER AND LIFE BECOMES EXCITING AND FUN.	FIXATES (FIXED MINDSET)	A FIXED MINDSET RESULTS IN LESS LEARNING AND FEAR OF MAKING MISTAKES, SO GROWTH IS LIMITED.
INSIDE (INSIDE GOALS)	INSIDE GOALS ARE MEANINGFUL AND SATISFYING. YEAH, YOU ENJOY IT WHEN OTHERS NOTICE, BUT YOU DON'T NEED IT.	OUTSIDE (OUTSIDE GOALS)	OUTSIDE GOALS ARE STRESSFUL BECAUSE YOU'RE ALWAYS WORRIED WHAT OTHER PEOPLE ARE THINKING. YOU TEND TO GIVE UP WHEN YOU DON'T GET REWARDED.

Don't worry, this is hard for everyone and many of us need to work on this superpower. Just remember to tune into your body for answers. If you feel lots of stress, ask why you're doing what you're doing. Try to get closer to Character Grows Inside and you'll feel much better. Your body doesn't know how to lie!

FEEL-GOOD INDEPENDENCE

Your body also talks to you about your blossoming independence. It can be confusing because you can feel resistant to doing certain tasks–studying, doing dishes, and cleaning your room. A typical reaction is to put off the task until tomorrow or next week, referred to as *procrastination*. When you put tasks off, they become even harder to do later. You may feel relieved when you get out of doing a task now, but it's still *you* that needs to do it later.

One of the reasons your body tells you, "Don't do that thing, it's too hard," is because your brain gets overwhelmed thinking about completing major tasks. So instead, break up the task into small steps. Or better yet, just start on it and see how far you can go. Maybe you choose to do it for five minutes but find once you get started, you can do more than you thought. Usually the task is not as terrible as your brain made it out to be (we love you brain, but sometimes you overreact).

Other times you might need help. So if your parents ask you to do the dishes but you feel like it's too overwhelming, be honest with them (this is too much mom, can you help me?). It's easy for school work to turn stressful. But this stress may simply be trying to tell you that you need a better system for keeping your work organized. Ask a family member to help you develop a system and structure for all your school demands, including keeping your room clean. Having a nice place to work, a system for keeping track of your studies, and a room that is free from distractions helps you focus and work better.

Here's the thing about being more independent with tasks around the house and in school. You'll take pride in yourself. Being independent feels great! Yeah, it takes work, but you'll feel a new level of confidence and control in your life. Your parents will appreciate it too and might even give you more say once you are contributing more.

LISTEN TO YOUR WISE VOICE

We all have a wise voice inside us. Often referred to as *intuition,* this quiet, inner voice helps to steer you throughout life. It's not quite the same as feelings and your Internal Compass. It's more like a wise, inner guidance system that draws you towards certain activities and people and away from others. It can be hard to hear this voice with the pressures and busyness of life. But the more you connect with yourself and give yourself space to listen, the stronger this voice becomes.

Nowhere does this voice have more of an impact than with doing what brings you joy. Having something in your life that excites you provides a sense of purpose. But you need exposure to different activities to find what you like. This is a great time to experiment with different activities and notice what gets your "juices flowing."

Some activities you try you'll love right away, and others take more time before you decide. Like playing an instrument isn't fun at first, but after you start to get the hang of it, your enjoyment increases. And why not try something your parents have been asking you to do? Remember, you don't have to be in a hurry to find activities you love, but if you never try, how will you know?

You want to listen to that wise voice about these activities. What gets you excited? Do your parents have to drag you to the activity or do you go willingly? Look for what experts call "flow," that feeling that you just lose yourself (and track of time) in what you are doing. This is a positive sign! Maybe you love a subject in school so much, you decide to join a club or activity.

Sometimes the voice doesn't make sense, like nudging you to learn more about music even when your family is not musical. Or trying theater when you've always been into sports. It knows things about yourself that you may not know yet and it's the icing on the cake of Super You.

SUPER ADVICE

Be on the lookout for hobbies! Hobbies include an element of learning such as reading, cooking, singing, gardening, art, listening to/playing music, collecting anything (baseball cards, dolls, rocks) or sewing. The great thing about hobbies is there are more ways to learn than ever. YouTube alone can teach you almost anything. Hobbies also give your life a sense of purpose and can even turn into a career one day (or not, it doesn't matter because they are so enjoyable).

TIME TRAVEL

When it comes to doing household chores and school work, time travelling ahead even a few hours can help. So before cleaning your room, imagine how you will feel when it's clean and orderly. Same with school work. Character Grows Inside may be harder now, but will make you happier in the future as you slowly become the person you were meant to be. Think about the amazing and unexpected things that will happen when you let your inner voice guide you. Time Travel to consider how excited you'll feel becoming Super You!

SUPER YOU IN ACTION!

Here are some examples of becoming Super You which can make you feel proud of yourself.

GETTING INDEPENDENT

Jen was an only child and her parents did everything for her. They told her as long as she did well in school and softball (her sport), everything would be taken care of for her. She didn't have to do chores or help with meals or anything. When Jen went to her friends' houses she noticed how they did more on their own. She felt a little envious at the independence they had, while she stayed dependent on her parents. Although she had plenty of time to focus on her studies, she felt something was missing.

After learning about the importance of independence, she used Time Travel to consider how feeling dependent on her parents would feel in her future when she goes away for college and lives on her own one day. Although it would make her life harder now, she asked her mom if she could do more around the house. Her mom was more than willing to let her take on a little at a time. Soon Jen was pitching in during meals and helping clean the house. She felt more confident and continued to do more at home.

TOO MUCH STRESS

Jackie loved tennis and did well in school but she often felt stressed about both. She worried she wouldn't win matches and put pressure on herself to get good grades. She was always worried she was getting someone mad at her.

Super Knowledge taught Jackie that outside goals were increasing her stress. She truly enjoyed tennis and liked school too.

Time Travel showed her that school would only get harder and so would the competition of tennis. So Jackie got into the habit of watching her stress level and then changing her focus from outside to inside goals. She focused on getting better at tennis, not winning. She focused on improving her study habits, not her grades. She found this inside goal focus helped her learn and enjoy life more. Plus, her stress went way down.

Fixed Mindset

Ever since Alison was little she knew she excelled at things. She read early, excelled in sports, and school came easy. As she got into middle school she could see other kids catching up. She still did well but was afraid to try new things for fear she would fail. She liked getting approval from her teachers and parents. Although she was tiring of soccer, everyone always complimented her on her skill. Her inner voice was pushing her to learn a musical instrument but she was deathly afraid to start at the bottom. She stayed safe with school and soccer and made a point not to try things she didn't know for sure she could succeed in.

After gaining Super Knowledge about a growth mindset, Alison realized she was giving up growth and learning for safety and approval. She tapped into her growth mindset superpower and inside goals. She acted on her wise, inner voice and started taking flute lessons. And those lessons gave her confidence to try out for band later in middle school, followed by band in high school, where she met lifelong friends and ended up majoring in music in college.

Outside Powers

Super You is about taking time to get to know yourself, the type of person you want to be, and learning to listen to that wise voice directing you to your future (super) self. In a world full of people, there's still only one Super You!

And we are off to the last section, which is all about learning about your outside powers. They are the finishing touches to growing a healthy body during puberty!

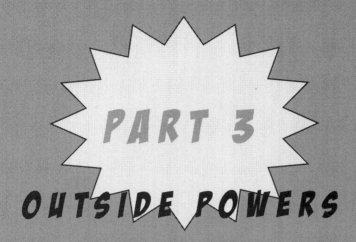

PART 3

OUTSIDE POWERS

"I EMBRACED WHO I AM, AND I DON'T WANT TO STOP."
- KARA DANVERS (SUPERGIRL)

CHAPTER 8

CRITICAL THINKING

YOU CAN MASTER YOUR PHYSICAL AND EMOTIONAL POWERS AND BOOM! The outside world challenges everything you learned. If you aren't careful this seemingly invisible force can deplete your powers. Luckily, you can fight back with your Outside Powers. And you do this by tapping into your amazing ability to think critically.

SUPER KNOWLEDGE: X-RAY VISION TO THE RESCUE AGAIN

Before you can think critically, you need to understand how culture plays favorites: the two worlds (virtual and real), and the nature of news.

WHEN CULTURE PLAYS FAVORITES

Every day you get messages from the culture about how you should look, what you should eat (and not eat), and who you should be. *Culture* is a collective idea about what is considered acceptable or good.

What I call "cultural faves" are specific preferences of a culture that aren't right or wrong. Every girl should become aware of cultural faves, especially when it comes to body type and shape. These preferences of culture change over time.

Consider that in the 1800s, plump and curvy women were considered the picture of beauty. Peter Rubens was a 17th-century famous Flemish painter known for his paintings of big, full-figured women. Because of his popularity, "Rubenesque" was a term to describe women who fit this ideal body type. In addition to curves, women also wore corsets, which is a garment laced tightly around the waist, used to create an hourglass figure.

In the 1920s, curves went out of style and "in" was having a flat chest, short, bobbed hairstyle, and a curve less, boyish figure. From 1930 to 1950, the curvy look came back (without the cinched waist). The most notable celebrity to embody this look was Marylyn Monroe. Having curves and large breasts was considered the ideal body type. There were even ads to help thin women gain weight.

In the swinging 60s it was in style to wear a mini-skirt and be tall and slim. Models like Twiggy became the preferred body shape. This didn't last too long, as in the 1980s the fit and toned look came in as health became more of a focus. But fast-forward to 1990 and "thin is in" returned with models like Kate Moss. The body shape preferred in women after 2000 was a bit of everything—fit, toned, and thin (but not too thin). At this time there is a small (but important) movement towards acceptance of people of all shapes and sizes.

Culturally acceptable female body types is always changing, and nowadays it favors more slender bodies than times past. The media's preferences for this is called the *Thin Ideal*. These trends have little to do with what is healthy or right for you as an individual.

A NOTE ABOUT REWARDS

Cultural faves come with real rewards in the form of attention. Just remember, striving to reach a cultural fave that isn't right for you will cause you more pain than reward. Cultural faves aren't just about looks; they also include personality, school, and family. In some areas, you'll fit into cultural faves and others, you won't. Being yourself will bring you the most internal rewards and that's what truly makes you happy.

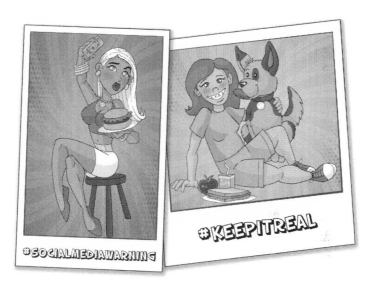

THE TWO WORLDS

Did you know you are a digital native? This is someone who was born into a technology-based society with smart phones and tablets. It's important to understand that you live in two different worlds: virtual and real. The virtual world is manmade and includes what you view online; but for this book I'm including TV, movies, and magazines. Real life is how things really are—often referred to as *realistic* or *reality*.

Understanding why the virtual world is different will help you critically think about it. Let's touch on a few differences here:

UNREALISTIC IMAGES

When you see a glamorous photo in a magazine, it's almost guaranteed that it's been touched up. Software like Photoshop removes blemishes and can make someone look thinner or larger and make skin appear smooth. Nowadays anyone can touch up their own photos with features on their phone or by installing an app.

A lot of the images you see also come from hours of work done by professional hair stylists and makeup artists. A hair stylist ensures that hair looks flawless and a makeup artist applies makeup for the sole purpose of making the wrinkles and blemishes disappear so that the pictures turn out perfect. In real life, most of us don't have someone doing our makeup and hair every day. In fact, if you were to spot a celebrity without her makeup on, you probably wouldn't recognize her.

ADVERTISING

You also view advertising while watching TV, going online, and from bloggers or YouTubers supporting a product. It's important to remember that the goal of advertising is to sell you a product. Advertisers do this by showing possible benefits like happiness, health, and well being.

For instance, females are often told a product will make them beautiful. Maybe it's a clothing brand, makeup or skin-care product, or even something about your weight and shape. You will see the person in the advertisement look beautiful and happy, perhaps surrounded by lots of friends.

Remember, like everything in the virtual world, ads are manmade and a lot of thought goes into them. They handpick models or actors, they digitally alter them to look better, and they film them a bunch of times until they get it right. They make things look as perfect as possible, including the product, so you will buy it.

SUPER TIP!

Be aware of food advertising! Fast food is shown as delicious and satisfying, and nutritious food as "healthy." And then there are the quick fixes." If you just take "this" or eat "that," you'll be healthy or able to change your body. For example, boys who want to grow muscles may see an advertisement for a protein supplement saying it can give them muscles, when in reality, puberty gives them muscles; and because boys grow later, they will just have to wait until it happens naturally.

SOCIAL NETWORKING SITES

Social networking sites are where people connect online by posting updates, photos, and messages. Most social network sites have a minimum age of 13, but not everyone follows these rules. If you don't have an account you may have seen your mom's or dad's accounts. Facebook, Instagram, and Snapchat are popular now, but this can change.

While it can be fun to keep up with people on social sites, what we see on social media may lead to bad feelings. We see pictures of the party we weren't invited to, or our friend's family is on a luxurious vacation our family can't afford, or we see people on the go doing fun things, while we're bored at home.

Although social media from friends is not the same as advertising, it's important to remember that people are choosey about what they post. For example, you may not know that your friend was sick the entire time on her vacation from the one photo posted (it's not cool to post pictures of puking!). Or you don't know that your friend's mom only allowed a few people to come to the party and that's why you were left out. Nobody posts pictures of themselves laying around in their PJs, which we all do once in awhile.

ONLINE CONNECTION DOESN'T REPLACE REAL-LIFE CONNECTION

Social sites don't replace the very real health benefits we get from "real life" human connection. So if you haven't ventured into this world of social networks, that's totally fine. And when you do (or if you are in it now), proceed with caution and realize it's just one way to keep in touch. If it becomes the only way, you'll miss the joy that comes from face-to-face interactions with other people.

PROMOTING STEREOTYPES

Be aware of the looks-orientated *stereotypes* you see on TV, videos, or in movies. A stereotype is an automatic association we make about someone based on how they look. For example, it's common for heavy women to be teased by men, followed by audience laughter. Children's shows often portray big kids as disliked and of poor character, like Harry Potter's greedy and mean cousin Dudley. On the flip side, princesses are seen as beautiful while wicked witches are shown as ugly.

Don't get me wrong, these stories can have important messages; but it's important to notice how looks-oriented stereotypes can develop. We may not even be aware of how the virtual world we visit affects our beliefs about people.

The problem with stereotypes is we make a judgment before we get to know the person for who they really are. So be on the lookout for unfair stereotypes so you don't fall prey to judging others based on what they look like. In other words, don't judge a book by its cover!

Table 8.1 reviews the key differences between virtual life and real life.

TABLE 8.1: THE DIFFERENCE BETWEEN THE TWO WORLDS

VIRTUAL LIFE	REAL LIFE
IT'S A MAN-MADE IDEA, TO LOOK A CERTAIN WAY AND EVERYTHING IS MADE TO SEEM EASY.	IT'S GOT A TON OF VARIETY AND IS MUCH MORE COMPLEX THAN THE VIRTUAL WORLD.
CONTAINS UNREALISTIC PHOTOS AND IMAGES WITH HAND-PICKED MODELS, PROFESSIONAL HAIR AND MAKEUP DONE, AND PHOTOSHOPPED TO TAKE AWAY IMPERFECTIONS.	FULL OF EVERYDAY LOOKING PEOPLE. MOST DON'T HAVE THEIR HAIR AND MAKEUP DONE UNLESS IT'S A SPECIAL OCCASION, AND PHOTOS REFLECT REAL PEOPLE.
PRODUCTS LOOK AMAZING AND THE ATMOSPHERE CREATED AROUND ADS MAKES YOU THINK IT WILL MAKE YOU HAPPY	SOME PRODUCTS ARE HELPFUL AND OTHERS ARE A DISAPPOINTMENT. ANY HAPPINESS THEY BRING IS SHORT-LIVED.

EVERYONE POSTS THE BEST PICTURES AND TIMES IN THEIR LIFE. SOCIAL MEDIA IS GOOD FOR KEEPING IN TOUCH; NOT SO GREAT AT CONNECTING.	REAL LIFE IS A MIX OF GOOD, NEUTRAL, AND CHALLENGING TIMES. FACE-TO-FACE INTERACTION MAKES US FEEL TRULY CONNECTED.
PEOPLE LOOK PREDICTABLE AND YOU ONLY SEE HAPPY ENDINGS (MOVIES CAN SUMMARIZE YEARS AND YEARS IN TWO SHORT HOURS).	PEOPLE COME IN ALL SHAPES AND SIZES AND LIFE IS FULL OF WINS, CHALLENGES, AND SETBACKS.

THE NATURE OF NEWS

No doubt you'll read headline news, articles, and blogs. The news uses dramatic headlines to catch our attention. Remember that journalists aren't scientists, so when they talk about research they often make it too simplistic—claiming certain foods (and bodies) are good or bad. Try not to read too much into the news headlines of the day; and if you have questions or are worried about something, ask your parents.

As you use the internet to do research for school projects, you need to understand that not all information you find is accurate. Anyone can start a blog and say this or that is healthy. Look for reputable websites and organizations that take all the research into consideration. Sites that end with a .org (nonprofit companies), .edu (associated with universities) and .gov (government sites) tend to be more credible than .com and .net.

When something sounds too good to be true (or too bad to be true), that's a red flag. For example, someone may go on about how immunizations cause health problems when research clearly shows they help people stay healthy and stop the spread of infectious diseases. Table 8.2 provides a list of red flags and good signs for the articles you read.

TABLE 8.2: HOW TO TELL IF IT'S CREDIBLE

GOOD SIGNS	RED FLAGS
CITES RESEARCH WHEN MAKING CLAIMS (MORE LIKELY TO OCCUR WITH .ORG, .EDU, AND .GOV)	MAKES CLAIMS WITHOUT CITING RESEARCH (CONSIDER GOALS OF WRITER WITH .COM OR .NET)
DISCUSSES HEALTH IN TERMS OF DIETARY AND ACTIVITY PATTERNS	CLAIMS ONE TYPE OF FOOD OR EXERCISE IS "GOOD" OR "BAD" FOR HEALTH
REASONABLE AND DOABLE HEALTH ADVICE LIKE WALKING MORE OR FITTING IN MORE NUTRITIOUS FOODS	EXTREME ADVICE, LIKE HAVING TO CUT OUT FOODS YOU LOVE OR DOING A CERTAIN TYPE OR CRAZY AMOUNT OF EXERCISE
INTERVIEWS EXPERTS THAT SHED LIGHT ON THE TOPIC	CLAIMS EXPERTS DON'T KNOW WHAT THEY ARE TALKING ABOUT
HEALTH FOCUSED	LOOKS FOCUSED

BODY TALK: FROM PASSIVE TO ACTIVE

Now that your mind has all the Super Knowledge and your X-ray Vision is intact, let's consider how to move from passively accepting the virtual world to being active in how you experience it.

TWO DIRECTIONS: BODY AND SELF-IMAGE

Messages and images from the virtual world can act like a mirror, influencing how girls and young women feel about their bodies and themselves. The term *body image*, relates to how you think and feel about your body and how others perceive it. *Self-image* is how you feel about your whole self.

Without the knowledge presented here, it's all too easy to passively sit back and accept what you are seeing. This passive viewing means girls judge themselves based on an unrealistic standard. That's because the mind doesn't know that these messages and images are unrealistic. So it feels threatened and can make you try to compete, which is no fun.

Body image became a hot topic over the last few decades as the negative effects of media images came to light. But it's been around longer than that. Consider this: How did women feel in the 1800s if they didn't have the full, "Rubenesque" figure? What about the popularity of thin and flat-chested flappers in the 1920s? How did full-figured gals with bigger breasts feel during that time? Or in the 1950s when Marylyn Monroe's body type was considered ideal? Slender women probably didn't feel so hot about how they looked.

The answer is not to try and be what the outside world says you should be. You should question these messages every step of the way. This is where you start to use all your superpowers. You know there's more to you than what you look like. You know your body has a genetic blueprint and that what you can control is how you take care of it. You don't need to look a certain way or buy something to love your body and yourself. As actress and writer Reema Zaman discovered: "*My turning point came when I realized that I am beautiful precisely as I am, and my "troublesome imperfections" are actually my complexity, and part of my authentic power. Complexity is what makes every human being unique, powerful, and inspiring, each in her own way.*" For her entire story see Super Advice.

SUPER ADVICE

Growing up as a girl born in Bangladesh and raised in an American school in Thailand, I felt constantly at war with my body, and with what the world considered "beautiful." It seemed that nearly every trait of mine—the color of my skin, my body type, the shape of my facial features, the texture of my hair, my intelligence, my imagination, my natural inquisitiveness, ambitiousness, and strong opinions—were seen as being unattractive, unladylike, unpopular, and undesirable. Every message from my parents, the popular kids at school, and TV, magazines, movies, and other media made me feel like I was the walking embodiment of troublesome imperfections. So I started to shrink myself down, physically, emotionally, creatively, and intellectually. I kept my voice tiny and timid, and made sure to silence my opinions. I reigned in my dreams and goals, and aspired for goals that were big but not "too big." My turning point came when I realized that I am beautiful precisely as I am, and my "troublesome imperfections" are actually my complexity, and part of my authentic power. Complexity is what makes every human being unique, powerful, and inspiring, each in her own way. Furthermore, I realized that if I wanted to make a true impact in the world, that impact would come from owning, celebrating, and living from my complexity. Our purpose in life is not to shrink; our purpose in life is to continually expand. By living as our fullest and truest self, we help others do the same. One by one, through our beautiful complexity, we can truly change the world.

— Reema Zaman is an award-winning author, speaker, and actress from Bangladesh

ONE OF YOUR MOST POWERFUL SUPERPOWERS: CRITICAL THINKING

We all venture into the virtual world and consume media, it's just a part of life. But doing so in a way that keeps you from developing limiting beliefs (like thinking you're not good enough) is vital. It's all about asking questions, thinking for yourself, and developing beliefs that are in line with your core values. The more you learn how to critically think about the multitude of media messages you receive, the happier and healthier you'll be

Critical Thinking is all about asking questions. When it comes to advertising ask yourself: Is this product as good as it looks on TV? Does it sound too good to be true? Is this advertisement instilling a belief that isn't in line with my values? Use your Critical Thinking skills to evaluate advertising to make sound decisions and keep limiting beliefs from developing.

Let's take food advertising as an example. You may notice that fast food is often described as "tasty." While nutritious food is described as "healthy." When asking if this is true and in line with what we believe, the answer is no (at least it is for me). I believe in balancing all food for nutrition and taste, but advertising tends to show food as extremes—either healthy or unhealthy.

When it comes to viewing music videos, magazines, advertisements, or even celebrities walking down the red carpet, ask yourself: Do these images look like the everyday people I see? Who will benefit from this? Who might be harmed? Do these images reflect real life? Remind yourself that media images are created by man and can impact people in a variety of ways.

When it comes to news, blogs, and social media, ask if the information is true. For articles that make strong claims about "this" or "that" being good or bad, they need to earn your trust by showing proof. And when your mind rushes to thinking someone on social media has it better than you, ask yourself "Is this true?" This reminds you that this person is only posting the positive parts of her life.

The movies and shows you watch will promote stereotypes about people based on looks. Again, be aware of this and spot it when it happens. Is this really how people are? What stereotype are they presenting here? Has this been my experience? This helps you realize that the media you consume has flaws and inaccuracies, allowing you to keep your beliefs and values intact.

It's so important to view this man-made virtual world through a thoughtful and questioning lens. Critically thinking about these messages is like learning to read in the virtual world. Check out the examples of questions to ask in Table 8.3 when consuming media in the virtual world.

TABLE 8.3: CRITICALLY THINKING ABOUT THE VIRTUAL WORLD

TYPE OF MEDIA	QUESTIONS TO ASK
IMAGES	IS THIS WHAT EVERYDAY PEOPLE LOOK LIKE? HOW HAS THIS IMAGE BEEN TOUCHED UP?
ADVERTISING	IS THIS PRODUCT AS GOOD AS IT LOOKS ON TV? DOES IT SOUND TOO GOOD TO BE TRUE? IS THIS ADVERTISING TRYING TO INSTILL A BELIEF THAT ISN'T IN LINE WITH MY VALUES?
SOCIAL MEDIA	DOES THIS PICTURE SHOW HOW THIS PERSON'S LIFE REALLY IS? AM I SPENDING TOO MUCH TIME ON SOCIAL MEDIA INSTEAD OF IN-PERSON INTERACTIONS?

TV SHOWS	DOES THIS SHOW DEMONSTRATE HOW PEOPLE REALLY ARE? WHO CREATED IT AND WHAT WAS THEIR INTENTION? WHAT STEREOTYPE ARE THEY PRESENTING HERE?
NEWS ARTICLES AND BLOGS	WHAT SIGNS SHOW ME THIS INFORMATION IS ACCURATE OR NOT?

TIME TRAVEL

Let's say you allow the virtual world to guide your decisions. Time traveling to the future shows you that you will not be yourself, you will be what this make-believe world tells you to be. You will become a slave to it, always feeling like you are falling short (because it's unrealistic and no one can live up to it). Being consumed by this means you miss out on your real life, the one you were meant to live. But if you, instead, live your real life on your terms, you will feel in control of your life. Yes, you will still visit the virtual world, but you are smart about it and it won't get you down, because you have learned to question it.

SUPER DECISIONS: CRITICAL THINKING IN ACTION

See how to use your Critical Thinking powers to manage both virtual and real life!

PHONE DRAMA

Piper had a cell phone for about a year. She texted her friends and got on Instagram once she turned 13. She spent a great deal of time on her phone. While it was fun at first, she started to feel lonely. She would be home on a weekend and see pictures of friends going out doing fun things. She texted her friends a lot but didn't see them much. She worked hard to make her life appear better on social media by taking photos when her family and friends did fun things. Even though she felt better when posting and getting likes, this didn't last long and so she did it even more.

When Piper gained Super Knowledge about the virtual world, she realized she was relying too much on social media to connect with others. Time Travel told her that no amount of likes would make her feel better in real life. So she made plans with friends, posted less, and re-engaged with life and the activities she enjoyed. And most of all, she regularly questioned the times she thought someone else's life was better than hers. After all, everyone posts their best moments on social media.

Media Comparisons

Isabelle was often online and enjoyed looking at teen magazines. She had her favorite movie stars and pop singers and loved to find out about their lives. Problem was, she started developing a poor body image when she compared herself to them. After gaining some Critical Thinking skills, she began asking questions. Is this what most people look like? What else is at work helping them look so glamorous? She began to understand that they were in a different world and many of the images were touched up. This helped her feel better about herself and her body.

Instead of passively accepting what she saw in the media, Isabelle questioned it. This helped her see it all in a more realistic light. She still had fun following her favorite stars, but stopped comparing herself to them.

FROM CRITICAL THINKING TO PRESSURE REDUCER

Critical Thinking is demanding and seeking evidence for what is presented as true. Without evidence, it's just another opinion. Now it's time to focus on the other daily pressures you'll experience and the power you have to reduce them.

CHAPTER 9

THE PRESSURE REDUCER

IT'S NOT JUST THE VIRTUAL WORLD THAT SENDS MESSAGES ABOUT health; so do the people you interact with day in and day out. It could be a teacher, a friend, an acquaintance, a coach, or a family member. It's important to be prepared for the world of opinions if you're going to honor your body's superpower. This is where you get to use your Pressure Reducer superpower. It's pretty cool!

SUPER KNOWLEDGE: RECOGNIZING PRESSURE

We all face pressures of daily life. If we're not careful, these pressures can turn you off to a healthy and happy life. Recognizing it is the first step.

WHAT IS PRESSURE?

We all feel *pressure* from the outside world. Pressure is defined as "an attempt to persuade or coerce (someone) into doing something." This can be a well-meaning adult telling you to eat your vegetables because they're "healthy." Your PE coach gets on your case because your mile time isn't improving. And your

English teacher insists you won't be successful unless you learn how to write well.

On the receiving end of pressure is resistance. You can think of it like a game of tug of war. One side is pulling and seems to be winning but then the next side pulls back. This is pressure and resistance. You're told what to do and come back with "I don't want to do it." And so the game of tug of war goes on.

Being praised for something can feel like pressure too. For example, if Suzie's teacher always talks about what a great student she is, Suzie might feel pressure to keep up her studies and not disappoint her teacher. It's important to remember that people doing the pressuring usually have good intentions.

But some of the worst pressure can be the pressure you put on yourself. As long as you stay hard on yourself, whatever you're trying to accomplish stays on the outside and never penetrates the inside where it can grow. In other words, it only adds to the resistance you feel. It also adds even more stress.

Unfortunately, many of the things you feel pressured to do can enrich your life. So the first step is to realize this problem of pressure happens to everyone. We all go out into the world and can let these pressures get us down.

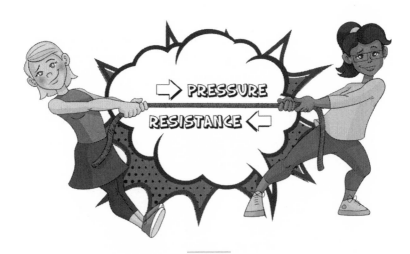

PRESSURE ABOUT BODIES

Pressure about bodies can be experienced in many different situations. And it can be indirect or direct. For instance, you may hear friends or adults say bad things about their body. They might make fun of a body part or call themselves fat. You might also hear them talking about other people and their bodies in a negative way.

The adults or friends in your life may put pressure on you about your body. They may directly mention their desire for you to have a lower weight or try to get you to diet. Even though the intention is usually to improve health or performance, the approach is not a recommended one. See chapter two for advice on how to handle outside advice.

This pressure can influence how you feel about your own body. Use your Critical Thinking superpower and question these messages. After all, research shows that when kids focus on weight and have a negative view of their body, they don't do as well in school, are more likely to become depressed, may not grow right, tend to exercise less, and eat fewer nutritious foods. Negative body talk does not make people healthier!

PUT YOURSELF IN YOUR BODY'S SHOES

Think how you would feel if you were being criticized all the time. That's how your body feels. When we are always saying negative things to our body about how it's not right, and this or that needs to change, it doesn't feel so hot. It works hard to keep you healthy, and this negative talk just brings it down.

A World of Nutrition Experts

Nutrition is one area that many people have many opinions on. But it's important to remember there is a difference between factual information (like a vitamin has a certain function in the body), and judgments or opinions.

As we discussed in Super Functioning, a nutritious diet is important throughout life, but especially during periods of rapid growth. But if someone says how a certain food like cookies or chips are "bad," that's an opinion. In reality food can't be bad; it's just how often we eat it that might be bad for us. If we have ice cream for every meal, that would be bad. These judgments can make eating less enjoyable, and people feel guilty about their choices, so just be aware of this difference.

For example, my son came home from kindergarten announcing that "ice cream makes you fat." That was an opinion he heard from someone at school; but it's not a fact, because no food has the power to change weight and size. In Appetite Signals we talked about how you eat as being important for helping your body grow the way nature intended. What you eat over time matters for your health; but the belief that a single food or food group can transform a body to be a different size is very common today.

Sometimes, information about an area of nutrition is emerging, meaning there's promising evidence, but more research is needed. People can take this information and make it seem like it's a fact when it's not. So be aware of the difference between fact, opinion, and emerging science as listed in Table 9.1

TABLE 9.1: DIFFERENT TYPES OF INFORMATION

FACTUAL	OPINION	EMERGING
I KNOW THIS INFORMATION IS TRUE BECAUSE THERE'S ENOUGH RESEARCH TO SUPPORT IT	I KNOW THIS INFORMATION IS OPINION BECAUSE IT'S BASED ON SOMEONE'S EXPERIENCE OR WORD OF MOUTH (MY FRIEND'S MOM SAID IT WAS TRUE!)	I'M NOT SURE THIS INFORMATION IS TRUE OR NOT YET. IT'S A NEW NUTRI-TION AREA THAT RESEARCH IS BEGINNING TO EXPLORE.
EXAMPLE: HOW VITAMINS AND MINERALS FUNC-TION IN THE BODY	EXAMPLE: YOU HEAR SOMEONE SAY: "I HEARD X IS BAD FOR YOU, AND PEOPLE SHOULD NEVER EAT IT."	EXAMPLE: WE KNOW HEALTHY GUT BACTERIA IS IM-PORTANT, BUT RESEARCH CAN'T SAY FOR SURE YET IF EVERYONE BENEFITS FROM TAKING BACTERIA IN THE FORM OF PROBIOTIC SUPPLEMENTS.

BODY TALK:
THE THREE PRESSURE REDUCER TECHNIQUES

Now that you know how pressure develops, let's get into the techniques that help you reduce it in your life so you can take action instead of relying on resistance. In other words, end the tug of war game!

1. DO A VALUE CHECK

Start with listening to your body. You may notice you feel resistant to something others want you to do. Let's take choosing an extracurricular activity as an example. Maybe you mentioned an interest in an activity to your mom and she signed you up without asking you. So you feel some resistance and dread going. Even though you had some interest before, when it was pushed on you, it changed the experience.

Outside pressure affects your *motivation* to do things. Motivation is your level of desire to do something. So when something feels like pressure, you don't want to do it, or you do it and it feels more stressful (low motivation). But when you really want to do something, it's much easier to do, minus the stress (high motivation).

We can't change every single person's reaction, but we can change our own. So catch yourself when you get into the mindset that you *should* do something. Remind yourself why you're doing it and how it will benefit you. This is what I call doing a value check. If it's school related, remind yourself of the importance of learning. If it's eating nutritious meals, focus on feeling good and giving your body what it needs. These activities are supposed to make your life better, so that is what you need to focus on.

And when it comes to the self-critical voice in your head, turn to your friend, self-compassion, because beating yourself up is the worst type of pressure there is. Instead of being hard on yourself, give yourself credit for what you have done. Realize that everyone struggles and give yourself a break. Talk to yourself like you would a close friend. Notice how this changes your motivation. I think you'll see that you're more productive and can more easily accomplish things.

2. MAKE THE SWITCH TO AN APPRECIATION MINDSET

We talked about negative body talk and why that doesn't help. But what can you do instead? You can practice appreciating your body. You just need to be aware of your mindset, which is the way you view and relate to your body. This is switching from what I call a "disapproving mindset" to an "appreciation mindset."

A disapproving mindset is focusing on all the ways your body falls short of fitting some ideal body type, which may be different for everyone. For example, someone short may want to be tall. And someone thin may want more muscles. And someone heavier may want to be more petite. Even though it seems like certain girls fit this ideal, they too can have a disapproving mindset about their body. Anyone can!

So catch the times you're judging your body and instead, think about what you appreciate about it. Remind yourself of all your body systems working hard to keep you healthy and functioning (e.g., seeing, walking, hearing, etc.). Think positive about your body and respect it, and it (and you) will be happier and healthier.

Here's one of the most important things you will learn in this book. Having a disapproving mindset doesn't change your body, but it does dampen all of your superpowers. It's harder to listen to Body Talk, your emotional powers don't work as well, and your mood goes down. But when you appreciate your body, it's easier to master its superpowers and that makes you more like you, which is all anyone could want. See table 9.2 for the difference between a disapproving and appreciation mindset.

TABLE 9.2: DISAPPROVING VERSUS APPRECIATION

DISAPPROVING MINDSET	APPRECIATION MINDSET
YOU FOCUS ON BODY FLAWS AND HOW YOU WANT TO CHANGE THEM ("I WISH I HAD...")	YOU NOTICE AND APPRECIATE YOUR BODY'S GOOD QUALITIES AND UNIQUENESS ("I LIKE THAT MY BODY...")
YOU DEFINE BEAUTY BY WHAT'S ON THE OUTSIDE ONLY ("I CAN ONLY BE ATTRACTIVE IF I LOOK A CERTAIN WAY.")	YOU DEFINE BEAUTY BY WHO YOU ARE AS A PERSON ("I FEEL LIKE I'M ATTRACTIVE EVEN THOUGH I LOOK DIFFERENT FROM WHAT I SEE IN THE VIRTUAL WORLD.")
YOU WEAR CLOTHES TO COVER UP YOUR BODY OR THAT DON'T WORK FOR YOUR BODY TYPE BUT ARE TRENDY ("THIS COVERS UP WHAT I DON'T LIKE ABOUT MY BODY.")	YOU WEAR CLOTHES THAT COMPLIMENT YOUR BODY AND REFLECT YOUR UNIQUE SENSE OF STYLE ("THIS ENHANCES MY BODY AND MAKES ME FEEL GOOD.")
YOU HAVE A NEGATIVE VIEW OF YOUR BODY BASED ON UNREALISTIC BEAUTY STANDARDS ("I'LL NEVER LOOK LIKE KATY PERRY.")	YOU HAVE A POSITIVE VIEW OF YOUR BODY BASED ON ALL IT DOES FOR YOU ("LOOK AT ALL THE THINGS MY BODY CAN DO.")
YOU FEEL UNCOMFORTABLE IN YOUR BODY BECAUSE YOU WISH IT LOOKED DIFFERENT ("I JUST DON'T FEEL RIGHT IN MY OWN SKIN.")	YOU FEEL COMFORTABLE IN YOUR BODY BECAUSE YOU ACCEPT IT AND GIVE IT WHAT IT NEEDS ("I FEEL GOOD MOST THE TIME, AND I CAN BE MYSELF.")
MAKES IT HARDER TO USE YOUR SUPERPOWERS AND YOU FEEL LIKE SOMETHING'S MISSING	EASIER TO USE ALL YOUR SUPERPOWERS AND YOU FEEL LIKE YOURSELF

3. FOCUS ON WHAT WORKS FOR YOU

You will hear lots of advice from others about nutrition. When you try to take this advice and apply it to your life you might feel that resistance again. And that can turn your motivation in the wrong direction. Plus, you can't be sure if the advice is on target.

Mostly, people tend to talk about what works for them, but that might not work for you. Just like there isn't one career path, there isn't one way to eat or exercise. You know you are on the right track with what you're doing if it *feels* right for you and you enjoy it.

So you may hear that running is the best form of exercise; but if you like to walk or play tennis, one of those would be the better choice *for you*. When your body enjoys eating and exercise, it gets more out of it. In fact, enjoying your food means your body absorbs more nutrients. Exercise shouldn't feel like work; it should be a release and something you look forward to.

There will be lots of opinions on nutrition out there that can increase pressure. Combat this by focusing on what works for you, because only you know how different foods make you feel and taste. Luckily, there isn't only one right way to eat, be active, and live your life.

TIME TRAVEL

Similar to Critical Thinking, living a life trying to please others is not a happy life. Look ahead and you can see yourself feeling stressed with a life that lacks true inner meaning. But by using your Pressure Reducer you can live the life you were meant to have, by living out your values, appreciating your body, and focusing on what works for you. It makes health and happiness a lot easier in the future, even though it takes courage right now.

SUPER DECISIONS:
THE PRESSURE REDUCER IN ACTION

Let's see how to use the three pressure-reducing techniques to live an (almost) pressure-free life!

VALUE CHECK

Victoria's mom really valued a clean house so she was always on her to keep her room clean. This always felt like pressure to Victoria. She felt she just couldn't enjoy her life because she always had to make sure her room was clean. The more her mom bugged her to clean, the less she wanted to, and it was a big problem between the two of them.

Super Knowledge made Victoria realize the tug of war that was going on and Time Travel told her that having a clean room would help her. In order to the reduce the pressure she was feeling, Victoria did a value check. She realized she could think better while doing homework when her desk was clear. She also liked it when her room was picked up and her bed was made. She actually valued having a clean space and reminded herself of that when her mom got on her. She even talked to her mom about allowing her to clean *before* nagging her, and they got along much better. She had a clean room *and* less pressure!

APPRECIATION MINDSET

Jody had two friends who hated how all their clothes looked on them and always complained that their thighs and stomachs were huge. This made Jody start to question her own body and whether or not it was right or good enough. Sure enough, she started disliking how she looked and had trouble finding the right clothes to cover herself up.

Super Knowledge helped Jody see what a disapproving mindset would do to her life, and she knew she wouldn't take very good care of her body in the future. So she made the switch to an appreciation mindset. She took the time to value all her body could do. She played basketball and appreciated her abilities. She also focused on what made her body unique and tried to give her body what it needed. She found clothes that showed off her sense of style and that fit her body well.

An appreciation mindset made a big difference and it took the pressure to look perfect away.

WHAT WORKS FOR YOU

Sydney's PE coach thought sugar was "toxic," so she challenged all the kids in her 8th grade class to go a week without sugar. Sydney tried, but by the end of the week she gave in and had ice cream. She felt guilty and even when the challenge stopped, she felt differently about sweets. She'd try to avoid them, but usually ended up eating too much, instead.

Super Knowledge taught her that these beliefs about sugar were just an opinion, not fact. If she kept this no-sugar diet up, she would end up eating lots of sugar and think about sweets all the time. Her teacher's beliefs about food didn't work for her. She decided to eat sweets and enjoy them, but not all the time (like she did before). This meant she didn't feel guilty and ate sensible amounts. When her coach talked about sugar, she no longer felt pressure or guilty, knowing she had made a choice that worked for her.

FROM PRESSURE REDUCER TO THE CONCLUSION

The Pressure Reducer is being able to identify pressure and reduce it with your values, appreciating your body, and focusing on what works for you.

You made it to (almost) the end of this book. I hope that learning about your physical, emotional, and outside powers has helped you become an expert on your body's superpower.

Next, I have summarized the nine superpowers that will help you all the way through adolescence and beyond.

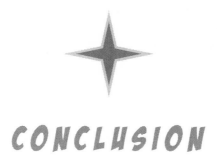

CONCLUSION

9 SUPERPOWERS FOR THE ADOLESCENT GROWTH SPURT

I HOPE YOU RE-READ THE BOOK AND PRACTICE YOUR SUPERPOWERS in a journal. Here's a place you can come to when you are feeling unsure about what do. By looking through this list—and asking the right questions—you can start figuring things out.

Do I understand everything that is going on with my body?
If you're feeling confused about what's happening during puberty, you may simply need to learn more or review what you've learned.

Superpower #1: X-ray Vision is learning about the changes going on in your body and accepting and using them to your advantage. You can also turn to all of the *Super Knowledge* sections for information.

I believe having solid information is important when making decisions. When we don't understand something fully, our mind doesn't have all the information it needs in order to make a wise decision. Understanding a subject helps you problem solve and figure out what you can and can't control.

Is my growth on track? I'm not sure.
If you're concerned with your growth or your hunger signals seem out of whack, start with Superpower #2: Appetite Signals. **Appetite Signals are about trusting your body's signals for food and giving it what it needs to grow the way nature intended.**

Your body needs a constant stream of nourishment and your Appetite Signals of hunger, fullness, satisfaction, and cravings are your body's way of telling you how much you need.

Am I getting the nutrition I need?
When your body talks to you in terms of feeling sluggish, constipated, or having stomachaches, you'll want to visit Superpower #3: Super Functioning. **Super Functioning is learning what your body needs during the adolescent growth spurt and applying nutrition into your eating so it's enjoyable and you feel great.**

Revisit this chapter and use the next section to help boost your nutrition in a way that works for you. You can also talk to your parents about meal planning.

Am I moving my body enough during the day so it feels good and full of energy?
When your body talks to you in terms of feeling tired or unmotivated, visit Superpower #4: Super Focus. **Super Focus is about identifying your body's exercise and sleep helpers and then putting them to work to sharpen your mind and life.**

This one can be hard because we don't always feel like being physically active. But it's the physical activity that gives us energy. Also, getting outside is good for us, so combining activity with the outdoors makes your body very happy.

Am I giving my body enough time to recoup with sleep?

If you're feeling sleepy at the wrong times of day, like during class, or if you feel very irritable and have trouble focusing, visit Superpower #4: Super Focus.

Getting enough sleep is important for everything in your life. When you fall short, you have trouble learning and may be in a bad mood. Read up on getting a sleep routine in place and honoring your circadian rhythm.

Am I dealing with the full range of emotions or am I trying to escape or avoid something difficult?

When unpleasant emotions come up, there can be a tendency to try to escape or avoid them. If you're feeling upset, angry, overstressed, sad, or are having difficulties in some area of your life, visit Superpower #5: Internal Compass. Internal Compass is discovering how your mind is developing and using your feelings and emotions to problem solve and live a better life.

Remember that when we don't let our feelings out or try to force them away, they stay inside and can cause problems. Also, not taking care of our physical health can make things worse.

Am I building and maintaining positive connections with others, or isolating myself?

If you find yourself alone often and feel something is missing, visit Superpower #6: Super Friends. Super Friends is acknowledging the importance of connection and being thoughtful when forming and maintaining friendships.

How are your connections going? You may have friends, but feel you can't be yourself with them. It may be time to branch out or start new activities which can bring you closer with those you have similar interests with.

Am I engaged with life, learning about myself and what excites me, or just going through the motions?

If you're feeling low on motivation and high on stress, visit Superpower #7: Super You. **Super You is about taking time to get to know yourself, the type of person you want to be, and listening to that wise voice directing you to your future (super) self.**

Maybe it's time to try a new activity, practice gratitude, check in with your mindset, or even be kinder to yourself. Remember that you are in the process of discovering yourself, so stop and see what else you could be doing differently.

Am I critically thinking about the virtual world or passively accepting it the way it is? How does this affect my "real" life?

If you're feeling down on yourself and perhaps your body, visit Superpower #8: Critical Thinking. **Critical Thinking is demanding and seeking evidence for what is presented as true. Without evidence, it's just another opinion.**

There are many virtual world messages coming your way about how to look and be. Without realizing it, these messages can make you feel like you're not good enough, decreasing body and self-image. Super Knowledge and Critical Thinking will help you move away from unrealistic standards in the virtual world.

Am I living out my values every day or letting outside pressures get me down?

If you're feeling pressure to reach a goal, be healthy, or enjoy your free time, visit Superpower #9: The Pressure Reducer. **The Pressure Reducer is being able to identify pressure and reduce it with your values, appreciation mindset, and focusing on what works for you.**

It's easy for anyone to let daily pressures get to them. The key is to reaffirm your values and be aware when this is happening. How you respond to pressure makes a big difference.

YOUR BODY'S SUPERPOWER

Together, these 9 superpowers make up *Your Body's Superpower*—a force for good not just in your life, but in the world. Going through puberty isn't easy; but real and rewarding growth never is.

More than anything, I want puberty to be an amazing transformation for you—one where you embrace your body and all of its amazing powers.

Now that you're a Superhero, go out into the world and practice your superpowers one small step at a time. Don't hesitate to come back here when you hit some bumps, which we all do. You can get over any challenge because you are strong, resilient, and unique. There's only one you, so let your light shine bright!

GLOSSARY OF TERMS

absorbed (absorption): The movement of substances into cells through a process called osmosis. This is what happens when nutrients are absorbed into the bloodstream from the digestive tract.

adolescence: The time period between puberty and adulthood. Early adolescence is roughly 10-14, middle is 15-17, and late is 18-21.

adolescent growth spurt: The rapid rate of growth in both height and weight that occurs during puberty.

appetite: The level of desire to eat and satisfy your body's need for food.

body image: How someone sees and feels about their body, what they believe about their appearance, and how they physically experience their body. Body image can be positive, negative, or neutral.

Bullying (all types): Using power negatively towards someone, which includes repeated aggressive or mean-spirited behavior. *Verbal bullying* uses words to make fun of or start rumors about someone. *Physical bullying* uses pushing, hitting, blocking or unwanted physical contact to intimidate someone. *Relational bullying* uses tactics to purposely exclude people from a group. *Cyber bullying* occurs online in the form of texts, tweets, and mean comments.

calcium: The most abundant mineral in the body that is important for health. Humans need calcium to build strong bones, especially during puberty and late adolescence.

carbohydrates: One of the three macronutrients that provide energy for the body and is made up of carbon, hydrogen, and oxygen. Carbohydrates are found in fruits, vegetables, grains, and dairy foods in the form of sugars, starches, and fibers.

character: The general pattern for how someone interacts with others and treats themselves. Good character is often aligned with traits like honesty, perseverance, respect, caring, responsibility, and maintaining these behaviors even when it's hard or no one is watching.

circadian rhythm: The brain's 24-hour clock that makes someone feel sleepy or awake at predictable times. Also referred to as the sleep/wake cycle.

circulatory system: The body system that includes the heart, blood vessels, and veins that circulates blood throughout the body.

community: A group of people living, working, or doing a particular activity in the same area.

cortex: The outer layer of major organs such as the brain (cerebrum).

craving: A strong desire for something such as a certain type of food or taste (sweet, salty, sour, etc.).

culture: A collective idea or specific values that are shared by a group of people. Also refers to beliefs, traditions, and social norms of specific groups of people.

DHA: A fatty acid (docosahexaenoic acid) that is a component of the brain, cerebral cortex, and retina (eye). It is found mostly in fatty fish like salmon and tuna.

dietary supplements: Capsules, tablets, powders, bars, or shakes that contain nutrients or ingredients that may be difficult to get though diet. Can include vitamins, minerals, protein, herbs, and other ingredients. Supplements are not regulated by the FDA, so be sure to check with a parent.

dieting: Restricting calories/energy in order to lose weight.

digestive system: Where food travels after it is eaten; includes the mouth, esophagus, stomach, small and large intestine, and anus, along with organs that help food digest. The purpose of the digestive system is to break food down into small enough parts for the body to absorb.

endorphins: Natural chemicals (hormones) in the brain released during exercise that make you feel good.

endoskeleton: Skeleton that is inside the body, deep within body tissues.

energy (calories): The calories in the food we eat and beverages we drink. Like cars need gas, humans need energy from food. In short, a calorie is a unit of energy.

estrogen: A group of sex hormones in the female body that support its development and maintenance. During puberty estrogen rises causing changes to breast, pubic hair, body composition, and eventually maintains a monthly menstrual cycle.

exoskeleton: Outside skeleton that acts as a shell for the body, supporting and protecting it.

extrovert: Somebody who is outgoing and gets energy from being around people.

fat (body): A storage system in the body that protects internal organs, is used as an energy source, and is needed to begin and maintain reproductive functions in females.

fat (dietary): One of the three macronutrients that provide energy for the body made mostly of carbon and hydrogen. Fat is found in both plant and animal foods. Plant foods include nuts, seeds, avocados, and vegetable oils. Animal foods that contain fat include butter, meat, and full- fat dairy.

fiber: A component of plant foods that cannot be digested. It helps food move through the gastro-intestinal tract and makes stools (poop) soft. Fiber is found in fruits, vegetables, whole grains, and beans.

fortified: Nutrients added to foods after processing. For example, some orange juice is fortified with calcium and vitamin D.

fullness: When the stomach is filled with food and extends, signaling it's time to stop eating.

genes: Units of hereditary that are transferred to a person from their biological parents. Genes determine traits like hair color, height, eye color, and when you start puberty.

genetic blueprint This is the general frame and shape the body will be after it's done growing.

ghrelin: A hormone that increases appetite.

growth mindset: the belief that you can do better at something with effort and practice.

hippocampus: Part of the brain's limbic system, responsible for long-term memory and emotional responses.

hormones: Substances in the bloodstream that instruct other cells in your body to take action.

hunger: An increasing desire to eat, resulting in uncomfortable sensations such as stomach rumbling.

hypothalamus: A small part of the brain that releases hormones which launch the onset of puberty.

integumentary system: The skin, hair, nails, and sweat that help keep harmful substances from entering the body. It also regulates body temperature.

introvert: Someone who tends to be reserved around others. They may still enjoy social activities, but often need time alone to recharge.

intuition: To understand something without conscious reasoning or having to think much about it.

iron: A mineral that carries oxygen in the hemoglobin of red blood cells to the rest of the body. Iron is in both animal and plant foods including meat, seafood, poultry, beans, grains, and greens (like spinach).

leptin: A hormone that suppresses appetite and regulates weight and fat storage.

limbic system: The structures of the brain that involve emotional and behavioral responses.

luteinizing hormone: A hormone that helps initiate and regulate sexual development.

macronutrients: Nutrients that provide energy, including carbohydrates, protein, and fat.

magnesium: A mineral that has many functions in the body. Important for energy production, muscle contraction, bone development, and normal heart rhythm. It's found in both animal and plant foods including nuts, seeds, avocados, grains, yogurt, and spinach.

melatonin: A hormone that regulates sleep.

menstruation: The monthly hormone-directed cycle females go through to prepare for a possible pregnancy. It includes normal vaginal bleeding when the uterus sheds its lining.

micronutrients: Vitamins and minerals that do not provide energy but have important functions in the body.

mindfulness: Paying attention in the present moment.

minerals: An inorganic substance found in the earth. People need small amounts of minerals from food for their body to function properly.

mood: An emotional state that can be positive, negative, or neutral and can occur for no specific reason.

motivation: The level of desire to do something.

muscular system (musculoskeletal system): A system in the body that consists of skeletal, smooth, and cardiac muscles that allow the body to move, circulate blood, and maintain posture.

myelin (myelination): A fatty substance that covers nerve fibers to quickly transport electrical impulses throughout the brain. Myelination is a process that makes brain communication more efficient, which occurs during adolescence.

nervous system: It consists of the brain, spinal cord, and nerve fibers. The brain tells the body what to do and the messages travel via the spinal cord and nerve fibers to the rest of the body.

peak growth period: The time during puberty where growth is fastest in terms of height, fat, bone, and muscle.

peak bone mass: The amount of bone tissue one has by the end of skeletal maturation, which occurs at the end of the teen years and early twenties.

potassium: A mineral that helps regulate the balance of fluids in the body as well as supporting nerve signals and muscle contraction. It's found in plant foods such as fruits, vegetables, grains, and animal foods such as dairy.

prefrontal cortex: The part of the brain that is involved with planning, decision-making, reasoning, and controlling impulses.

premenstrual syndrome (PMS): The time before your period when estrogen decreases, resulting in moodiness along with other symptoms like pimples, bloating, feeling tired, headaches, and food cravings.

pressure: An attempt to get someone to do something you want them to do, or trying to talk ourselves into doing something.

probiotics: Live microorganisms that confer health benefits to the body. Food sources include yogurt, kefir, and fermented foods like sauerkraut.

procrastination: Putting off a task you need to do now because it is perceived as unpleasant.

protein: One of the three macronutrients that provides energy and builds and repairs body tissues. It is made up of amino acids. It's found in animal foods such as chicken, red meat, pork, and dairy and plant foods including soy, beans, nuts, and seeds.

puberty: The time period when the body gradually transforms from that of a child to an adult in terms of sexual maturity.

pubic hair: Coarse hair that grows around the vaginal area.

rapid eye movement (REM): A deep sleep when the eyes move in a jerky fashion.

satisfaction (meal): High enjoyment of eating that is followed by a low desire to eat again.

self-image: How you view yourself and your abilities.

skeletal system: The body system that acts as a structure for the body and includes bones, cartilage, and ligaments.

social networking sites: Online destinations where people post pictures, make comments, and gather followers/friends to show what they are doing in their life.

stereotypes: The automatic association people make about someone based on how they look.

testosterone: The primary sex hormone that is responsible for the development of male reproduction.

Thin Ideal: The media's preferences and glorification of thin, female bodies.

vaginal discharge: Fluid and cells shed through the vagina that keep it healthy. The consistency can be cream-like and sticky or clear and watery.

values: What is most important to people.

vegetarian: Primarily eats plant-based foods and excludes meat or animal products. Lacto-ovo vegetarians don't eat meat but do eat dairy products. Vegans exclude all animal products. And pescatarians eat fish.

vitamins: Organic compounds needed in small amounts by the human body for growth and nutrition.

vitamin A: A vitamin needed for vision, the immune system, and reproduction.

vitamin C: A vitamin needed for making collagen, enhancing the immune system, and metabolizing protein.

vitamin D: Fat-soluble vitamin needed for calcium to be absorbed and deposited into bone. It also plays many more roles in the body.

zinc: A mineral found in cells throughout the body. It plays a key role in growth and development and helps keep the immune system strong.

FOOD, RECIPE & MEAL MAKING IDEAS

Now is the perfect time to experiment with food and learn how to build snacks and meals. Just be sure you have supervision from an adult when using appliances for the first time.

We have ideas for incorporating more SUPER foods, featured recipes, and meal-making ideas.

SUPER IDEAS

Stick with fruits and vegetables at most meals and snacks. They are crunchy and make a great addition to any meal or snack

- fruit with breakfast or topped on cereal
- yogurt parfait with granola, honey and fruit
- peanut butter and banana sandwiches (or toast bread and top with peanut butter and sliced banana)
- side salad with lunch and dinner
- cooked veggies mixed in pasta with favorite sauce
- raw spinach on sandwiches instead of ice berg lettuce
- raw chopped veggies dipped in ranch or hummus

FEATURED RECIPE: HEALTHY SMOOTHIE
(submitted by Alora Koutnik)
Makes 2 servings

INGREDIENTS:

- 1/2 cup almond milk (or any milk)
- 3 tablespoons Greek yogurt
- 1 banana
- 1/2 cup frozen kale
- Half a carrot, not peeled (cut the end off)
- 1/2 cup frozen mixed berries
- 1/2 cup frozen strawberries

DIRECTIONS:

Mix in blender until smooth. Enjoy!

U*p calcium-rich foods where you can.* This includes dairy, non-dairy alternatives, and other foods that contain calcium.

See the calcium list to include different sources of calcium with your meals and snacks. The recommended amount of calcium for girls 9-18 is 1300 mg per day.

FOOD TYPE/PORTION	CALCIUM (MG)
FORTIFIED READY-TO-EAT CEREALS (¾-1¼CUPS)	137-1000
PARMESAN CHEESE, HARD (1.5 OZ.)	503
YOGURT, VARIETY (8 OZ.)	383-452
VARIETY OF CHEESES (1.5 OZ.)	287-430
ALMOND MILK (1 CUP)	451
TOFU, PREPARED WITH CALCIUM SULFATE (½ CUP)	434
ORANGE JUICE, CALCIUM FORTIFIED (1 CUP)	349
SOYMILK (1 CUP)	340

RICOTTA CHEESE, PART SKIM (½ CUP)	337
SARDINES, CANNED IN OIL, DRAINED (3 OZ.)	325
MUSTARD SPINACH (TENDER, GREEN), RAW (1 CUP)	315
MILK, VARIETY (1 CUP)	276-305
SALMON, CANNED WITH BONE (3 OZ.)	212
COLLARDS/SPINACH, FROZEN, COOKED (½ CUP)	145-178
COTTAGE CHEESE (1 CUP)	138
SOYBEANS, GREEN, COOKED	130
FROZEN YOGURT (½ CUP)	103
WHITE BEANS, CANNED (½ CUP)	96
KALE, FROZEN, COOKED (½ CUP)	90
ALMONDS, DRY ROASTED (1 OZ.)	76
CHINESE CABBAGE, RAW (1 CUP)	74
KALE, RAW, CHOPPED (1 CUP)	24
BROCCOLI, RAW, CHOPPED (½ CUP)	21

Pick whole grains half the time. These are unrefined grains such as oats, whole wheat bread, brown rice, and quinoa.

- Make sandwiches with whole wheat bread.
- Try oatmeal for a satisfying and filling breakfast.
- Use whole wheat/oat flour when baking muffins, waffles, and pancakes
- Include cereals that contain whole grains (look for the Whole Grain Council stamp on the package!)
- Try side dishes made with whole grains like brown rice, quinoa, and barley.

Eat fats too. Especially plant fat sources such as nuts and seeds, nut butters, avocados, and olive oil (they contain magnesium and vitamin E).

- For that crunch, add nuts and seeds to yogurt, cereal, and smoothie bowls.
- Top bread with nut butters like peanut butter, almond butter, or sunflower seed butter.
- Nut butters are also great for dipping (using apples or crackers).
- Cook and sauté food with olive oil.
- Make a vinaigrette dressing with olive oil to use for salads.
- Add wheat germ and/or flax to smoothies and baked goods.
- Add sliced avocado to sandwiches and eggs. See guacamole recipe to use on taco night or with some tortilla chips as a snack.

FEATURED RECIPE: EASY GUACAMOLE

INGREDIENTS:
- 1 medium avocado
- 1 Tbsp. plain yogurt
- 1 Tbsp. salsa
- salt, to taste
- lime juice (from a small squeeze of half a lime)

DIRECTIONS:
Remove the avocado pit and spoon the avocado into a small bowl and mash with yogurt and salsa. Add salt to taste and a just a bit of lime.

Realize the power of protein. Round out meals with a protein source. Aim to include fish and beans a couple of times a week.

- Include protein sources at most meals.
- Make sandwiches with turkey, tuna salad, or nut butters.
- Try beans and/or tuna in salads.
- Have hard boiled eggs on hand for a quick protein source to have with snacks or in the morning for breakfast.
- Make easy burritos with pinto beans, cheese, and flour or corn tortilla. Top with salsa and/or guacamole.
- Experiment with different ways to eat fish and try to have it two times a week. See the following recipe.

FEATURED RECIPE: SALMON NUGGETS

INGREDIENTS:
- 1 pound wild caught salmon (other fish will work)
- 1 egg
- 1 Tbsp. butter, melted
- ½ cup bread crumbs
- ½ cup Parmesan cheese
- ½ tsp. garlic powder
- ½ tsp. salt

DIRECTIONS:

1. Preheat oven to 400° F. Cut fish into 1-1.5-inch pieces.
2. In a small bowl mix the bread crumbs, Parmesan cheese, garlic powder, and salt. In another small bowl beat the egg and add the melted (microwave for a few seconds).
3. Dip each piece into the egg-butter mixture, roll in bread crumb mix, and place on baking sheet.
4. Bake 8-10 minutes or until cooked all the way through. Serve immediately.

BUILDING MEALS AND SNACKS

Building meals and snacks is easy, using food groups. Snacks can contain 1-3 food groups and meals, 3-5.groups. Discover your favorite combinations to increase nutrition and satisfaction!

FOOD GROUP	FOOD TYPE
FRUITS	APPLES, PEARS, BANANAS, BLUE-BERRIES, RASPBERRIES, HONEYDEW, WATERMELON, GRAPEFRUIT, GRAPES, PRUNES, PLUMS, DRIED FRUIT
VEGETABLES	CARROTS, CAULIFLOWER, BRUSSELS SPROUTS, SWEET POTATO, CUCUMBER, ZUCCHINI, SQUASH, MUSHROOMS, TOMATOES, GREEN BEANS, SUGAR SNAP PEAS, CELERY

GRAINS	WHITE: WHITE BREAD, WHITE RICE, BAGELS, CRACKERS, PRETZELS AND PASTA WHOLE GRAINS: OATS SUCH AS OATMEAL, POPCORN, CRACKERS, WHOLE CORN, WHOLE GRAIN PRETZELS, PASTA, AND BREAD, BROWN RICE, QUINOA
DAIRY AND NON-DAIRY SOURCES OF CALCIUM	MILK, CHEESE, YOGURT, COTTAGE CHEESE, NON-DAIRY ALTERNATIVES SUCH AS SOY, ALMOND, AND RICE MILKS
PROTEIN FOODS	ANIMAL SOURCES: BEEF, MEAT, PORK, CHICKEN, FISH, AND SHELLFISH PLANT SOURCES: BEANS, SOY, NUTS, AND SEEDS
FAT SOURCES	OILS, BUTTER, AVOCADOS, NUTS, SEEDS, AND NUT BUTTERS

HERE ARE SOME IDEAS:

SNACK IDEAS:
- Crackers (grain), cheese (dairy), and raw veggies with dip (veggies)
- Cookies with milk (dairy) and apple slices (fruit)
- Yogurt (dairy), nuts (fat/protein), and chopped berries (fruit)
- Carrot sticks (veggies), hummus (protein), and pita chips (grain)

BREAKFAST IDEAS:

- Egg sandwich (grain and protein) with chopped fruit (fruit)
- Pancakes (grain) topped with berries (fruit) with milk or yogurt (dairy)
- Yogurt parfait – yogurt (dairy), chopped nuts (protein/fat), and granola (grain)
- Whole grain cereal (hot or cold) (grain), with milk (dairy), and raisins (fruit)

LUNCH IDEAS:

- Sandwich with deli meat (protein/grain), tomato and lettuce/spinach (veggies)
- Green salad (veggies) with grilled chicken (protein) and a roll (grain)
- Quesadilla or burrito with beans (grain/protein), cheese (dairy) and veggies
- Pizza using flat bread or whole wheat English muffins (grain) topped with mozzarella cheese (dairy) and any other toppings (pepperoni, mushrooms, green peppers, etc.)

RESOURCES AND REFERENCES

A book with this much Super Knowledge takes a lot of research. Instead of filling up this book with references, I've listed them on my website at MaryannJacobsen.com/Super-Knowledge.

Here is a list of related resources that may be helpful to you:

BOOKS

The Care and Keeping of You: The Body Book for Younger Girls by Valorie Schaefer

Celebrate Your Body (And It's Changes Too!) by Sonya Renee Taylor

The What is Happening to My Body? Book for Girls by Lynda Madaras

The Intuitive Eating Workbook for Teens by Elyse Resch

The Self-Compassion Workbook for Teens by Karen Bluth

APPS

Magic Girl Period Tracker

The Human Body by Tinybop

Headspace (meditation app)

Three Good Things (A Happiness Journal)

WEBSITES

https://kidshealth.org/

https://www.girlsontherun.org/

https://charactercounts.org/

http://mediasmarts.ca/

https://beautyredefined.org/

https://biglifejournal.com/

https://www.raddishkids.com/

https://kidscookrealfood.com/

ACKNOWLEDGEMENTS

A book like this is only possible when many people come together. Thanks to the girls and moms who read the manuscript and provided feedback. Your time and honesty is much appreciated. And an extra special thank you to Lily Raymes for coming up with the title *My Body's Superpower*. That title inspired me more than you'll know. I loved being able to include words of wisdom from Marnie Goldberg, Jennifer Schmitt, Irina Gonzalez, Xian Horn, and Reema Zaman. Your stories will help many girls. And I'm grateful for Jill Castle, Karen Koenig, Emma Wright, and Karen Diaz for reviewing the book on a professional level. Your feedback was invaluable. And an extra special thanks to Karen Koenig for educating me about feelings, which was the impetus behind the Internal Compass chapter. Continue doing the amazing work you're doing. I always appreciate the hard work of my line editor/proofreader, Arnetta Jackson, who makes my writing much better. And I am especially grateful for Hannah Patrico for illustrating the cover while still in school (her mom Lisa Patrico instigated it all!). Your talent will take you far. Finally, is my family who puts up with me writing books. I'm sorry for those mornings I'm supposed to be making breakfast but you find me in the computer room writing and revising. And to Dan, my husband and financial advisor, you know I couldn't do any of this without you. I love you.

ABOUT THE AUTHOR

Maryann Jacobsen, MS, RD, is a registered dietitian, independent author, and mom. Through her unique writing style, Maryann empowers families to create a healthy relationship with food utilizing evidence-based strategies. She is co-author of

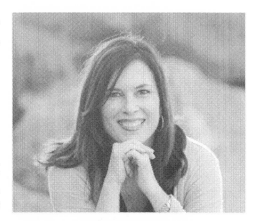

Fearless Feeding: How to Raise Healthy Eaters from High Chair to High School and author of *How to Raise a Mindful Eater* and *From Picky to Powerful.* She is founding editor of Raise Healthy Eaters (now MaryannJacobsen.com) and runs The Healthy Family Podcast. Her writing has appeared in the New York Times, Los Angeles Times, Mindbodygreen, and She Knows. As a family nutrition expert, Maryann has been quoted in various publications including *Parents, Scholastic Parent & Child* and *American Profile* and has been featured on *Good Morning America.* Find out more at MaryannJacobsen.com.

PRACTICE YOUR SUPERPOWERS

WITH THE COMPANION JOURNAL

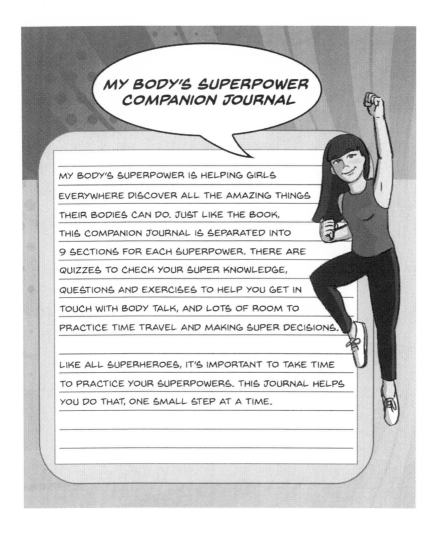

COMING SUMMER 2019

Made in the USA
Monee, IL
04 May 2020